Parasites and Human Disease

W Crewe
Reader in Parasitology,
Liverpool School of Tropical Medicine

and

D R W Haddock
Senior Lecturer in Tropical Medicine,
Liverpool School of Tropical Medicine

Illustrated by S M Crewe

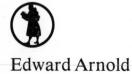

Edward Arnold

© W. Crewe and D.R.W. Haddock 1985

First published in Great Britain 1985
by Edward Arnold (Publishers) Ltd
41 Bedford Square
London WC1 3DQ

Edward Arnold (Australia) Pty Ltd
80 Waverly Road
Caulfield East 3145
PO Box 234
Melbourne

British Library Cataloguing in Publication Data

Crewe, W.
   Parasites and human disease.
   1. Parasites diseases
   I. Title
   616.9'6   RC119

   ISBN 0-7131-4473-4

Text set in 10/11pt English Times Compugraphic
by Colset Pte Ltd, Singapore.
Printed and Bound in Great Britain by Richard Clay (The Chaucer Press) Ltd, Bungay, Suffolk.

Preface

Parasitic diseases have always been a major cause of human suffering, and their effects have sometimes markedly influenced historical events. Even today parasitic diseases are among the most important causes of human morbidity. There are, for example, some 300 million people infected with malaria and 1.3 billion people infected with *Ascaris* in the world. Fortunately for the inhabitants of temperate countries, most of the serious parasitic infections of man are restricted to tropical and sub-tropical parts of the world. The parasites causing malaria, filariasis, leishmaniasis, trypanosomiasis and schistosomiasis are spread by vectors that are unable to survive in colder climates. Other parasites have life-cycles with free-living stages that also require warm climates for their survival.

There are, however, some serious parasitic infections which can be transmitted in temperate climates. The commonly held view that parasitic infections are uncommon in man outside the tropics is largely unjustified, and is based on the fact that the subject is rarely discussed privately or in print. Furthermore, the diseases in question are not normally reported, and therefore official statistics often contain no references to them.

There are many indigenous parasites in countries such as Great Britain, and many more 'tropical' diseases are imported in people coming from endemic areas. It must be remembered that one can travel half-way round the world in a day — a period well within the incubation period of most parasitic diseases — so visitors can easily 'import' parasitic infections into new countries. In addition many thousands of new residents, who may be infected with parasites, currently live in non-tropical countries.

A relatively small number of these parasitic infections can be passed on in the new countries, and so could become public health problems rather than just a matter of concern for the infected individual who brought in the disease. Most of them are transmitted by contamination of food and water, and in general their spread is restricted by the relatively high standards of personal hygiene in "developed" countries. Some parasites, however, may require more specific control measures.

In many of the warmer parts of the world, prevention of the spread of infectious diseases basically depends on improvements in socio-economic conditions, improvements in standards of hygiene, and the provision of better housing, water supplies and education. These, unfortunately, are frequently beyond the financial capabilities of the countries concerned.

Possible means of controlling parasitic diseases are many, but opinions differ as to which are the most useful. Treatment of human or animal carriers of infection is important, and occasionally eradication of animal reservoirs of disease has been suggested. However, great difficulties obviously arise if the animals concerned are wild, not domesticated. One valuable method of control is to interrupt the route of transmission by controlling vectors (if there are any), or protecting susceptible individuals by physical defence against arthropod bites, by chemoprophylaxis or by immunisation. Human immunisation against parasitic disease is, however, still in the development stage. Early detection of infection, and treatment of infected individuals to prevent the serious effects, and spread, of infection is important. In some instances mass treatment of a population has been resorted to.

Parasitic diseases differ from (say) bacterial diseases in that the causative organisms can rarely be cultured and so are more difficult to find when present in small numbers. Also, the treatment required is often very specific and so it is necessary to make a precise diagnosis. There are few equivalents of the 'broad spectrum' antibiotics for the treatment of parasitic diseases.

The increase in world-wide travel and migration is making it steadily more important for groups such as general medical practitioners, hospital doctors and workers in diagnostic parasitology laboratories to realize that 'tropical diseases' can now be met in any country, to be able to recognize and identify such infections, and to be aware of any possible public health significance. However, the medical curriculum is now so crowded that there appears to be little time for the consideration of parasitic diseases and their pathology during undergraduate education, and postgraduate instruction on the topic is limited. For reasons such as this, diagnostic pathologists also may have had little training in parasitology, and be in need of guidance in this field. And finally, even those who have had some training in the past should be made aware of the considerable advances that have been made during the last decade in our knowledge of the diagnosis, fundamental immunology and therapy of tropical parasitic disease.

The purpose of this book is to outline important aspects of parasitic diseases, with emphasis on the biology and transmission of the parasites concerned, on laboratory and clinical diagnosis, and on therapy. Attention is also drawn to those medical conditions that are likely to affect people from the tropics arriving in temperate areas.

It is hoped that the book will help medical practitioners, laboratory workers and students to understand and diagnose parasitic infections, and assist the first group in treating patients with these infections. The book should also serve as an introductory text for individuals intending to work in warm climates.

General reading

Crewe W (ed.). *Blacklock and Southwell: A Guide to Human Parasitology*. 10th ed. London, Lewis: 1977.

Donaldson RJ. *Parasites and Western Man*. Lancaster: MTP Press, 1979.

Gilles HM. *Recent Advances in Tropical Medicine, No. 1*. Edinburgh, Melbourne and New York: Churchill Livingstone, 1984.

Knight R. *Parasitic Disease in man*. Edinburgh: Churchill Livingstone, 1982.

Manson-Bahr PEC, Apted FIC. *Manson's Tropical Diseases*. 18th edn. London: Baillière Tindall, 1982.

Marsden P (ed.). Intestinal parasites. *Clin Gastroenterol* 1978; 7: 1–243.

Strickland GT (ed.). *Hunter's Tropical Medicine*. 6th ed. Philadelphia: Saunders, 1984.

Warren KS, Mahmoud AAF. *Tropical and Geographical Medicine*. New York: McGraw-Hill, 1984.

Contents

David Haddock died before this book was completed, and before he was able to finish his revision and correction of the text; any errors and inaccuracies are therefore mine. I miss not only his expertise, but also his cheerfulness and help.
To David, a friend, this book is dedicated.

W. Crewe

Part I

Protozoal infections

Protozoa are single-celled animals. Superficially, a protozoan cell resembles a single cell of a higher animal, but the protozoan cell has highly developed organelles which enable it to carry out all the necessary activities of the cell such as feeding, locomotion and reproduction.

There is no generally agreed classification of the protozoa, but the four main groups in which parasites of man are found are usually referred to as the Sarcodina, the Mastigophora, the Ciliophora and the Sporozoa. These groups can basically be distinguished by their organelles of locomotion.

The Sarcodina, or amoebae, move by means of pseudopodia, which are temporary extensions of the cytoplasm. The remainder of the cytoplasm then flows into the pseudopodium, and in this way the animal changes its position; only rarely does an amoeba move progressively from one place to another. The Mastigophora, or flagellates, move by means of one or more flagella, which are whip-like organelles which beat to and fro and push or pull the protozoan through the medium in which it lives. The Ciliophora, or ciliates, move by means of cilia, which are short and hair-like and usually cover the whole surface of the protozoan. The cilia propel the animal by beating rhythmically. All these three groups of protozoa include both free-living and parasitic forms. The Sporozoa, however, are all parasitic. Those parasitic in man are intracellular parasites, and correspondingly they have no organelles of locomotion and show little capacity for translatory movement, except sometimes in the sexual stages of the life cycle.

1

Intestinal protozoa

The protozoa that live in the intestine of man include members of all four main groups of parasitic protozoa. Those from the first three groups normally live in the lumen of the intestine; the sporozoan parasites live in the cells of the intestinal walls.

Included in this chapter for convenience are a small number of protozoan parasites that live in parts of the body other than the intestine. These include the parasites that cause toxoplasmosis, primary amoebic meningoencephalitis and pneumocystosis.

The Sarcodina

The members of the Sarcodina, the amoebae, move by means of pseudopodia, which are temporary cytoplasmic processes thrown out from the body. The pseudopodia are used both for locomotion and for capturing food. Movement of the body caused by pseudopodia is known as amoeboid movement. The cytoplasm of an amoeba is usually differentiated into an outer ectoplasm and an inner endoplasm, but even when present this differentiation is not always obvious. The endoplasm contains the nucleus, food vacuoles and various granules. Most members of the Sarcodina have a single nucleus.

Reproduction is asexual, usually by simple binary fission in the active or trophozoite stage, and resistant cysts are commonly formed when conditions are unfavourable. The amoebae that are parasitic in man usually form cysts which are passed in the faeces, and by which the infection is transmitted. Only one species of intestinal amoeba, *Entamoeba histolytica*, is definitely pathogenic in man.

Entamoeba histolytica

This amoeba has a world-wide distribution, but is chiefly important in the tropics and sub-tropics. The trophozoites mostly occur in the large intestine of man, but they may occasionally invade the liver, and rarely invade other parts of the body, where they give rise to amoebic abscesses. The unencysted trophozoite is a small mass of cytoplasm, capable of amoeboid movement; its size varies considerably, but it is usually about 20 μm in diameter.

The single spherical nucleus is bounded by a thin limiting membrane on which are small grains of chromatin arranged in a regular pattern, and in the centre of the nucleus is a larger granule called a karyosome. The nucleus is not easily seen in the living amoeba. The endoplasm also contains many food vacuoles, in

3

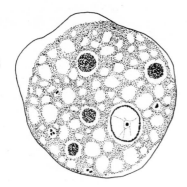

a. *Entamoeba histolytica*

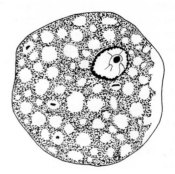

b. *Entamoeba coli*

c. *Endolimax nana*

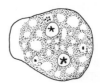

d. *Dientamoeba fragilis*

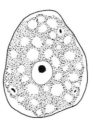

e. *Iodamoeba butschlii*

5μm

Fig. 1.1   Intestinal Amoebae. Appearance of trophozoites stained with haematoxylin.

which are various ingested particles such as bacteria, starch granules, faecal fragments and sometimes erythrocytes (Fig. 1.1a) *E. histolytica* is the only amoeba parasitic in man that ingests red blood cells.

When the trophozoite is about to encyst the cytoplasm becomes rounded and all inclusions are ejected. This rounded stage is known as the precystic stage, and it secretes the cyst wall. The cyst is spherical (occasionally ovoid) in shape, refractile, pearl-grey in colour, surrounded by a definite wall, and about 12 μm in diameter. The newly formed cyst has one nucleus, and contains food supplies in the form of a vacuole containing glycogen (the 'glycogen mass') and usually a number of rod-like structures known as 'chromidial bars' or 'chromatoid bodies'. There are usually two chromidial bars, but occasionally there may be only one, or several. The nucleus and the glycogen mass are not normally visible in the unstained cyst, but the chromidial bars may be visible as refractile blunt-ended bodies. As the cyst grows older the nucleus divides, and the glycogen mass and chromidial bars are used up and gradually disappear. The mature cyst contains four nuclei (Fig. 1.2a, b).

The cysts remain alive outside the body for only a few days in the faeces, but they can survive for much longer periods away from the faeces in suitable conditions. They cannot withstand desiccation or high temperatures. When the fully developed cyst, with four nuclei, is ingested by man the cyst wall is digested in the alimentary canal and the contained quadrinucleate amoeba emerges. Nuclear division then occurs, and the amoeba divides into eight uninucleate amoebae which grow and multiply by binary fission.

After a period of growth and multiplication in the intestine, encystment occurs and the cysts are passed out with the faeces. Unencysted amoebae may also be passed out, but these survive for only a short period, and even if ingested by man would be killed by the gastric secretions. Some strains of *E. histolytica* invade the mucous membrane of the large intestine and multiply there. Occasionally they may enter the portal blood vessels and be carried to the liver. Cysts are not formed in the liver abscesses, nor outside the body.

The acute stage of the disease is characterized by abdominal pain, and the passage of frequent diarrhoeic stools containing active amoebae, blood and mucus. During the chronic stages of the infection these symptoms disappear, and only cysts are found in the faeces.

Entamoeba hartmanni

Apart from a size difference, this parasite is very similar to *E. histolytica*, and until recently was usually referred to as the 'small race' of *E. histolytica*. However, because of certain morphological differences, particularly in nuclear structure and in the arrangement of the glycogen vacuole in the cyst, and because the 'small race' is not pathogenic, this parasite is now considered to be a separate species, *E. hartmanni*. The important differential character is that in the nucleus of *E. hartmanni* the chromatin granules on the nuclear membrane are few, large and irregular, while in *E. histolytica* they are numerous, small and regularly arranged.

The life-cycles of *E. histolytica* and *E. hartmanni* are similar. *E. hartmanni* is smaller than *E. histolytica* in both the trophozoite and encysted stages. The sizes

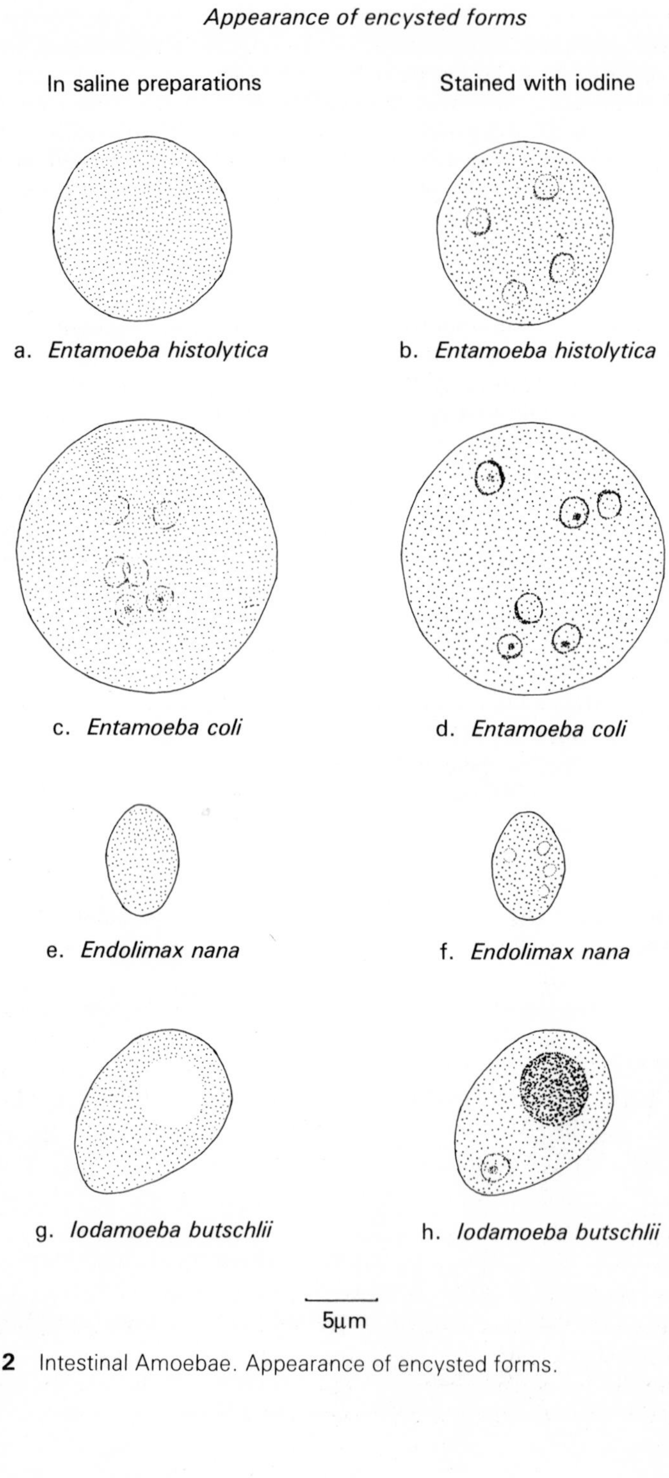

Appearance of encysted forms

In saline preparations   Stained with iodine

a. *Entamoeba histolytica*   b. *Entamoeba histolytica*

c. *Entamoeba coli*   d. *Entamoeba coli*

e. *Endolimax nana*   f. *Endolimax nana*

g. *Iodamoeba butschlii*   h. *Iodamoeba butschlii*

5μm

Fig. 1.2   Intestinal Amoebae. Appearance of encysted forms.

of amoebae, however, vary considerably with nutrition (*E. histolytica* from intestinal ulcers are about twice the size of those living in the lumen of the gut and feeding on bacteria and other particles), so the size of the trophozoite is not a reliable characteristic; however, the cysts of *E. hartmanni* measure about 6–10 μm and those of *E. histolytica* and 10–15 μm, so they can usually be distinguished. The presence of ingested erythrocytes is the only routine laboratory method of distinguishing unencysted forms of the pathogenic *E. histolytica* from those of the non-pathogenic *E. hartmanni*.

Entamoeba coli

Like the other species of *Entamoeba*, this parasite is world-wide in distribution; it occurs in the large intestine of man. The unencysted trophozoite is similar in size to that of *E. histolytica*, being about 20 μm in diameter, but the differentiation between ectoplasm and endoplasm is less marked, and the ectoplasm can usually be seen only when a pseudopodium is being formed (Fig. 1.1b). The endoplasm contains the nucleus and food vacuoles, but never erythrocytes. The nucleus is similar to that of *E. histolytica*, but the chromatin granules on the nuclear membrane, and the karyosome, are coarser than those of *E. histolytica*. This coarser nucleus is more easily seen in living specimens than is the nucleus of *E. histolytica*.

The cysts are about 18 μm in diameter, and when fully developed have eight nuclei which are more visible in unstained cysts than are the nuclei of the encysted *E. histolytica* (Fig. 1.2c, d). Chromidial bars are rarely present, but if present they appear as a bundle of fine rods. A glycogen mass is present in the younger cysts, but is not visible in unstained specimens.

E. coli is not pathogenic. It does not invade the intestinal mucosa, nor does it produce ulcers or liver abscesses, but otherwise its life-cycle is similar to that of *E. histolytica*.

Endolimax nana

This parasite is world-wide in distribution, although its prevalence varies in different parts of the world. It lives in the lumen of the large intestine of man, and also occurs naturally in monkeys. It feeds on bacteria and faecal fragments, and never invades the tissues of the host. It is a small amoeba, measuring only 6–12 μm in diameter (Fig. 1.1c). The ectoplasm cannot be distinguished from the endoplasm except when pseudopodia are being formed. The pseudopodia are few, short and blunt, and movement is sluggish. The nuclear membrane is usually free of chromatin granules, and the karyosome is large and irregular in shape. The food vacuoles contain bacteria, moulds and other particles but never erythrocytes.

The cyst is usually ovoid, about 8 μm × 6 μm, and is at first uninucleate; the nucleus then divides into two, then into four. The four nuclei tend to congregate at one end of the cyst, and the karyosomes become eccentric. The nuclei, however, are usually not clearly visible (Fig. 1.2e, f). The immature cyst contains glycogen which usually disappears before the cyst becomes mature. There are no chromidial bars. The mature quadrinucleate cyst is passed with the faeces and can survive outside the body for several weeks in suitable conditions. Infection occurs when the mature cyst is swallowed by man.

Iodamoeba butschlii

This is another harmless commensal, with a world-wide distribution. The trophozoites live at the base of the intestinal crypts, and so are rarely seen. Similar parasites occur in pigs and monkeys. The trophozoite is 8–12 μm in diameter, and resembles a small *E. coli*. Movement is sluggish, and there is no clear differentiation between ectoplasm and endoplasm except in the pseudopodia. The endoplasm is highly vacuolated, the food vacuoles usually containing bacteria but never erythrocytes. The nucleus is relatively large, with a large karyosome about half the diameter of the nucleus, and there are no chromatin granules on the nuclear membrane (Fig. 1.1e). In the space between the karyosome and the nuclear membrane is a layer of refractile globules.

The cyst is uninucleate, about 8–12 μm in diameter, and irregular in shape; it may be spherical, oval or pointed at one end (Fig. 1.2g, h). The nucleus of the cyst differs from that of the trophozoite because the granules congregate at one pole and the karyosome is forced into contact with the nuclear membrane. The glycogen mass is large and has a sharp margin, and it stains densely with iodine; it is this character that gives *Iodamoeba* its name. The glycogen mass does not disappear as the cyst matures, but it is largest in young cysts. Chromidial bars are not present.

Dientamoeba fragilis

This parasite is probably not a true amoeba, but the amoeboid stage of a flagellate closely related to *Histomonas*. It is world-wide in distribution, but generally considered to be rare in man. The trophozoite is small, measuring about 8 μm on average, and lives in the intestine of man and some monkeys, feeding mainly on bacteria. The nucleus is nearly always double (Fig. 1.1d), but rarely uninucleate forms may predominate. The trophozoite has a poorly defined ectoplasm and a granular endoplasm, and shows active progressive movement. The endoplasm contains many food vacuoles, but never erythrocytes. The nuclear membrane is thin and delicate, and has no chromatin granules. The karyosome consists of six large granules forming a star-shaped cluster, and it has been suggested that these granules are chromosomes, and that the binucleate condition represents an arrested phase of mitosis.

Trophozoites that are passed in the faeces degenerate very quickly. The cytoplasm first becomes frothy and vacuolated, the vacuoles then coalesce, and the degenerated amoeba is very difficult to recognize. This may partly explain the low recorded prevalence of this parasite in fresh faecal specimens. The cysts are not known, and the method of transmission is doubtful. It has been suggested that the infective stages of *D. fragilis* may be carried in the eggs or larvae of the threadworm *Enterobius*.

Free-living and coprozoic amoebae

Several species of free-living amoebae have been recorded in human faeces. These amoebae are widespread in soil and water, and probably are all (or nearly all) contaminants of the faeces. However, some free-living amoebae appear to be capable of invading mammalian tissue, and human infections of the eyes, lungs, sinuses, ears and central nervous system have been described. Infections of the central nervous system may lead to primary amoebic meningoencephalitis, and over 120 cases have been reported throughout the world during the past 20 years. Infections of other parts of the body are extremely rare, and are not usually serious.

The aetiology of the infections is unclear, but they are often associated with swimming in small bodies of warm fresh water that have been contaminated by sewage. The causative organisms are probably species of *Naegleria* and *Acanthamoeba*.

Medical aspects of amoebiasis

Pathogenesis

In most human infections with *E. histolytica* the amoebae are commensals, living in the lumen of the gut and causing no symptoms in their hosts. These people pass infective cysts. A proportion of asymptomatic cyst passers (possibly 25 per cent) have antibodies to *E. histolytica*, suggesting present or previous invasion of the tissues. A minority have illness due to tissue invasion. Some workers believe that pathogenicity is associated with a limited number of strains or 'zymodemes' of *E. histolytica*, e.g. II and XI identified by isoenzyme studies of enzymes produced by morphologically identical *E. histolytica*. Factors associated with a lowering of host resistance are caused by corticosteroid administration, cytotoxic drugs, neoplasia, AIDS, in late pregnancy or the puerperium, and with concurrent *Trichuris* infection. It has been estimated that, in Mexico, of every 1000 people with lumenal amoebiasis 200 have invasion of the intestinal wall and one will develop liver abscess.

When *E. histolytica* invade the intestinal wall they produce membrane damage and cytolysis by release of membrane-bound cytolytic enzymes. It has also been found experimentally that a cell-free extract of *E. histolytica* produces a cytopathogenic protein in tissue cultures and a factor destructive to polymorphonuclear leucocytes. Localized degranulation and destruction of these leucocytes may contribute to tissue destruction, endothelial damage, and thrombosis in capillaries and venules in the lamina propria. The trophozoites migrate into the crypts of Lieberkühn and destroy mucosal cells by proteolysis. The amoebae proliferate in the mucosa and in severe cases penetrate the muscularis mucosa and even the peritoneum. Flask-shaped ulcers with overhanging edges are produced. A central area of necrosis is produced with a low-grade inflammatory reaction; relatively few intact polymorphs are present. If there is secondary bacterial infection there will be a more acute inflammatory reaction. Fibrosis is usually minimal in all amoebic pathology, but occasionally a fibrous stricture of the gut results after healing.

The commonest sites of large intestinal infection are in the caecum, flexures, descending colon and rectum. Sometimes the ileum and appendix are involved. In severe cases the large intestine shows numerous deep ulcers with sloughs; in fulminant cases the whole mucosa will appear dark and gangrenous. Chronic granulomatous masses may form around the colon — these are called amoebomata.

Amoebic trophozoites probably metastasize quite frequently to the liver but in only a minority of instances cause amoebic abscesses. These are usually single, but sometimes two or more abscesses are found, most commonly in the right lobe. Essentially areas of necrosis and liquefaction are produced, the walls being made up of necrotic tissue and compressed liver parenchyma containing a cellular infiltrate with monocytes, plasma cells, lymphocytes and fibroblasts. Rarely the abscess is surrounded by a thick fibrous wall. The abscess may directly extend to surrounding areas including the pleura, peritoneum, intestines and pericardium (left lobe abscesses) and the skin. The perianal skin may also be invaded, and less commonly blood stream spread occurs to the lungs and rarely the brain.

Penile and cervical amoebiasis is a not uncommon problem in Papua New Guinea.

Immunity and host resistance

Severe invasive amoebiasis is much commoner in infections acquired in tropical countries than in those contracted in temperate climates. This may be partly due to variations in the virulence of the organism. Host factors which predispose to invasive amoebiasis include pregnancy, immunosuppression and possibly protein deficiency. In anaemic milk-drinking Masai, iron deficiency may have some protective effect which is lost on treatment with iron.

An attack of invasive intestinal amoebiasis does not protect against further attacks. Humoral antibodies are found in 90–100 per cent of those with amoebic liver abscess and 10–40 per cent of asymptomatic cyst passers, but they do not appear to be protective. It is believed that cell-mediated immunity, as indicated by lymphocyte transformation by amoebic antigens, is significant in host resistance to amoebiasis; studies in the Gambia suggest that lowering of host immunity may be necessary for establishment of invasive amoebiasis, and that possession of cell-mediated immunity may protect some of the population against amoebic disease.

Clinical features

The incubation period is usually 1–3 months, but it can vary from four days to several years. Abdominal symptoms should not be attributed to amoebiasis if only cysts are found in the stool.

Invasive intestinal amoebiasis

There is considerable variation in the severity of the illness. Often there is mild and intermittent diarrhoea with passage of four to six bulky, foul-smelling stools daily. The stools usually contain some blood and mucus. Colicky pains are experienced in the right and left iliac fossae. The pelvic colon and caecum may be tender on palpation. Bouts of diarrhoea characteristically last 1–3 weeks with some constipation during remissions. Constitutional signs are not prominent, though the patient may have a low fever. If the condition persists the victim loses weight and becomes anaemic.

In some cases the onset is more abrupt and diarrhoea is severe with tenesmus. There are febrile symptoms — the illness resembles bacillary dysentery of moderate severity. In these patients the liver is often slightly enlarged and tender; this is a 'toxic' hepatitis as seen in other inflammatory bowel diseases and is not due to direct amoebic invasion of the liver. Amoebic liver abscesses are very unlikely to develop during acute dysentery. Rarely invasive amoebiasis is fulminant with the rapid onset of severe diarrhoea, haemorrhage, shock and a tender distended abdomen in a gravely ill patient. There is considerable likelihood of colonic performation and peritonitis. The condition resembles toxic dilatation of the colon seen in ulcerative colitis, and the prognosis is poor.

Complications of intestinal amoebiasis

Local complications include:

1. peritonitis due to penetration or permeation of the gut
2. pericolic abscess
3. formation of amoeboma, a chronic granuloma around some part of the colon, which forms a palpable mass — it may cause intestinal obstruction or intussusception and can mimic carcinoma, diverticulitis or appendix abscess
4. appendicitis
5. extension of amoebic infection to the perianal skin
6. severe rectal haemorrhage
7. occasionally a condition of post-dysenteric colitis resembling ulcerative colitis, persisting for months after elimination of the parasite
8. stricture of the colon (this is unusual).

Distant complications include:

1. amoebic liver abscess
2. infection of pleura, lung or pericardium
3. occasional infection of other sites, including the brain, bladder, cervix, vagina, penis and spleen.

Amoebic liver abscesses

Amoebic liver abscesses can occur months or years after leaving infected areas. About half the patients will give a history of amoebic dysentery and most will not be excreting amoebic cysts in their stools. The disease is much more common in men than in women.

The onset is usually gradual, but can be acute. Pain over the liver area is the commonest symptom; this may be aching in nature but is often pleuritic in type with exacerbation by coughing. In a few patients diaphragmatic irritation causes right shoulder tip pain. A dry cough is often present. Patients sometimes notice a swelling in the right hypochondrium.

General symptoms include fever which may be swinging, nausea and vomiting. As in any chronic infective condition, anorexia, loss of weight, weakness and anaemia may ensue. If neglected the abscess expands with worsening symptoms, and localized extension leads to rupture on to the skin or into the peritoneum, pleura or pericardium. Less commonly gut, stomach, vena cava and right kidney may be involved by direct extension.

Physical signs include tenderness over the liver, either below the costal margin or in the lower intercostal spaces. The liver is palpable below the right costal margin, or in the epigastrium if the left lobe is involved. In advanced cases there will be bulging or pointing of the abdominal or chest wall when the abscess is about to burst.

Chest signs are associated with upward enlargement of the right lobe of the liver and include diminished movement of the right lower chest, dull percussion note in the right lower chest anteriorly and posteriorly, and diminished breath sounds in the right lower zone. Sometimes signs of a right-sided pleural effusion are present.

Jaundice is found in only 5–10 per cent of cases but is not deep — it is due to obstruction of bile ducts.

Amoebiasis in children

Amoebiasis is often considered a disease of adults but in fact is frequent and tends to be more acute in children especially when malnourished and following measles. Liver abscess is more fulminant and in contrast to adults has an equal incidence in males and females.

Clinical diagnosis of amoebiasis

Intestinal amoebiasis
Intestinal amoebiasis should be considered a possibility in patients from endemic areas with chronic or relapsing diarrhoea, passage of blood and mucus in the stool, colonic masses, and acute dysentery. It should not be forgotten that cosmopolitan conditions such as carcinoma of the large bowel, ulcerative colitis and intestinal tuberculosis occur in tropical areas, and indeed amoebiasis may be superimposed on carcinoma of the colon. Amoebiasis must be excluded before treating any tropical resident with corticosteroids as these drugs may convert a latent infection to an invasive one. Sigmoidoscopy can aid diagnosis by identifying characteristic amoebic ulcers with fairly normal intervening

Table 1.1 Causes of dysentery or diarrhoea

'Dysenteric conditions' that may all cause colitis	Shigellosis
	Campylobacter infections
	Schistosoma mansoni infections
	Balantidiasis (rare)
	Ulcerative colitis (rare in tropics)
Chronic or relapsing diarrhoea	Giardiasis
	Irritable gut syndrome
	Malabsorption
	Crohn's disease
Passage of blood and/or mucus in the stool	Carcinoma of the large bowel
	Haemorrhoids
	Diverticulitis (rare in tropics)
Presence of pericolonic mass	Carcinoma of the colon
	Ileocaecal tuberculosis
	Appendix abscess

mucosa and in obtaining scrapings for microscopy. Sigmoidoscopy should not be carried out in the severely ill patient with extensive colonic involvement as perforation can result. A barium enema is not very useful except for exclusion of other disease such as neoplasia. In general, parasitological diagnosis is essential. Conditions that need differentiation from intestinal amoebiasis are shown in Table 1.1.

Amoebic liver abscess
Differential diagnoses include conditions that cause (a) a tender enlarged liver with or without jaundice, (b) pyrexia of uncertain origin with or without clinically enlarged liver, and (c) pathology at the base of the right lung.

Common differential diagnoses are:

1. primary hepatoma (prevalent in tropical areas); kala-azar (associated with splenomegaly and leucopenia); virus hepatitis; pyogenic liver abscess; hydatid cysts; leukaemia; cirrhosis of liver; heart failure;
2. malaria (liver often palpable); tuberculosis; reticulosis; enteric fever (liver may be palpable);
3. right lower lobar pneumonia; right basal effusion.

In amoebic liver abscess, chest X-ray and screening of the lungs often shows an elevated right hemi-diaphragm and diminished movement of the right diaphragm. Ultrasound examination and radio-isotope scanning are useful in detecting the presence and site of fluid-containing liver masses and the response to treatment.

The polymorphonuclear count is usually elevated in ALA and serological tests for amoebiasis are nearly always positive. Liver function tests such as transaminases are not usually abnormal, but the bilirubin and alkaline phosphatase may show slight elevation. Aspiration is not essential or desirable for diagnosis but may be needed if pyogenic liver abscess is suspected. If diagnostic facilities are limited a therapeutic trial of metronidazole is reasonable.

Management of amoebiasis

The objectives are elimination of the parasite, relief of symptoms, correction of pathophysiology and prevention of recurrence. The following drugs may be effective:

(1) Metronidazole (Flagyl) is active against *E. histolytica* in the tissues, gut wall, liver and to a lesser extent in the intestinal lumen. It is relatively non-toxic but can cause anorexia, giddiness, vomiting and lassitude. Intravenous and rectal suppository preparations are available for seriously ill patients. Alcohol must be avoided during metronidazole therapy.

Intestinal amoebiasis — 2 g orally in one dose daily for 3 days or 800 mg 3 times a day for 5 days followed by diloxanide furoate (Furamide).

Hepatic amoebiasis — 800 mg 3 times a day for 10 days is recommended followed by diloxanide.

(2) Diloxanide furoate 500 mg 3 times a day for 10 days is active against *E. histolytica* in the gut lumen and less so against those in the tissue wall. It is used as sole agent in cyst passers and following metronidazole in invasive intestinal disease and hepatic amoebiasis. Toxic effects are mild but include occasional

flatulence, vomiting, urticaria and pruritus. Many other drugs have been used; some are mentioned briefly below.

(3) Tetracyclines are not directly amoebicidal but are used with metronidazole when there is severe intestinal disease with worry about perforation. Gentamycin is also used.

(4) Dehydroemetine is a tissue amoebicide, is cardiotoxic but less so than emetine, and is given by subcutaneous or intramuscular injection in daily doses of 1.5 mg/kg (maximum 90 mg) for 5 days in intestinal amoebiasis and up to 10 days in hepatic amoebiasis. It is useful for the occasional case which does not respond to metronidazole.

(5) Di-iodohydroxyquinoline is an amoebicide effective in the intestinal lumen in doses of 650 mg 3 times a day for 20 days.

(6) Chloroquine is moderately effective in hepatic amoebiasis in doses of 300 mg base daily for 20 days (with metronidazole).

(7) Tinidazole is very similar to metronidazole and may be used in its place with an adult dosage of 2 g daily for 3 days and 50–60 mg/kg per day in a single dose for children. It may be less likely to cause gastro-intestinal upset than metronidazole.

Indications for treatment

All cases of invasive amoebiasis need treatment. The treatment of asymptomatic cyst passers is more controversial. A high percentage of the population may be passing cysts in tropical areas — investigators found that over the course of a year 98 per cent of the population in some Gambian villages passed cysts. If it becomes feasible easily to identify pathogenic zymodemes, treatment might be restricted to patients passing these parasites. At the moment the following cyst passers should probably be treated: (a) those who have left endemic areas, (b) food handlers, (c) those being treated with corticosteroids, (d) those with a history of recurrent dysentery, and (e) possibly pregnant women. In practice many cyst passers if identified as such are treated.

General remarks on treatment

Intestinal amoebiasis
Metronidazole and then diloxanide are used in the doses indicated above. Loperamide (Imodium) may be given briefly for a day or two to control diarrhoea before the amoebicides work. Tetracycline or gentamycin is used if there is suspicion of peritonitis or in severe cases. In peritonitis surgery is hazardous, and reliance may be placed on suction, intravenous fluids and antibiotics. Repair or resection of a colon that has generalized disease is difficult. Some advocate temporary ileostomy and peritoneal drainage. Relapses are common. Stool examinations should be repeated at 1, 3 and 6 months.

Liver abscess
Aspiration for therapeutic purposes is not performed routinely, but it is if the abscess seems about to rupture, is very large or if response to treatment is poor. A large bore needle with stilette and 3-way tap is used. The best place for aspiration may be indicated by ultrasound; if this is not available the site tried is any bulging or area of maximal tenderness. If these cannot be clearly defined,

try the ninth intercostal space in the anterior axillary line to a maximum depth of 9 cm. No more than two attempts should be made — if unsuccessful, surgical drainage is indicated.

Amoebomas
These usually respond to the standard antiamoebic therapy and tetracycline, but are sometimes resected when mistaken for carcinoma or if causing obstruction.

Amoebic brain abscess
This seems to be almost always fatal — fortunately, it is rare.

Fulminant (necrotic) amoebic colitis
This is a serious condition requiring parenteral amoebicides (metronidazole and dehydroemetine) and antibiotics, gastric suction, intravenous fluids and possibly blood. Peritoneal drainage and ileostomy may be needed.

Primary amoebic meningoencephalitis

Pathology

The organisms probably gain entry to the cranial cavity through the nasal passages, cribriform plate and fibres of the olfactory nerve. They produce a diffuse leptomeningitis and inflammation of the superficial parts of the brain, particularly the base of the brain, medulla, frontal and temporal lobes and cerebellum.

Clinical picture and diagnosis

The incubation period following exposure to infected fresh water when bathing is 1-9 days. There may be an onset with upper respiratory symptoms and blocked nostrils followed by a rapidly evolving meningitis picture with headache, neck stiffness and mental confusion, going on to coma and death in a few days.

Diagnosis is from bacterial and viral meningoencephalitis, and lumbar puncture is essential as soon as possible to identify the pathogenic agent.

Treatment

Several drugs have been tried in therapy with little success. Amphotericin B in a dose of 1 mg/kg per day by intravenous infusion appears the most promising.

Laboratory identification of intestinal amoebae

Actively moving trophozoites of amoebae are found only in diarrhoeic stools. Normally the amoebae encyst as they pass down the intestine with the faeces and emerge with the faeces as cysts, but when diarrhoea is present they are passed out before encystment. Diarrhoeic stools may also contain cysts (they may, in fact, contain any stages of any of the protozoa in the gut lumen), but normally cysts are passed in formed faeces.

Identification of trophozoites

There are various factors, such as temperature and the freshness or otherwise of a specimen of faeces, which greatly affect the motility and general appearance of unencysted amoebae. If the stool is perfectly fresh and is examined on a warm stage, any amoebae present will be seen moving actively and extruding pseudopodia. Macrophages found in stools are about the same size and may easily be mistaken for amoebae; but macrophages do not show active pseudopodial movement and have a large obvious nucleus. Although the different species of human parasitic amoebae differ in size, this is not a reliable characteristic and is of little value in diagnosis. Similarly, the nuclei of different species are different, but examination of nuclear detail requires fixation of the faecal smear and staining with haematoxylin, and would not normally be attempted in routine laboratory practice. It is therefore very difficult to identify the species of amoebic trophozoites by morphological characters. However, the only amoeba which it is normally important to recognize in the unencysted stage is *E. histolytica*, the only one pathogenic to man. In acute amoebic dysentery a proportion (often a high proportion) of the trophozoites of *E. histolytica* passed with the diarrhoeic faeces will contain ingested erythrocytes — and only when erythrocytes are identified in a moving amoeba can a sure diagnosis of acute amoebic dysentery be made.

In acute amoebic dysentery the trophozoites of *E. histolytica* should be found fairly readily, moving actively and progressively if the preparation is from a freshly passed stool. The number present in any preparation is a matter of chance, depending from which part of the intestinal lesion the blood and mucus has come. There may, for example, be hundreds of amoebae in a low-power field, or only a few in a whole coverslip preparation. Active *E. histolytica* show little differentiation between ectoplasm and endoplasm. The nucleus is usually invisible, and the cytoplasm granular and vacuolated. These large trophozoites measure 10–30 μm, and if they contain ingested erythrocytes they are identifiable as *E. histolytica*.

In subacute amoebic dysentery loose stools without blood or mucus may be passed. Those stools may contain smaller amoebae, about 12 μm in size, with vacuolated cytoplasm, and with the nucleus visible in some individuals. These amoebae do not show the same rapidity of movement as the large trophozoites. They are the so-called 'precystic amoebae', and it is not possible to identify them specifically without staining.

Identification of cysts

Many structures of cyst-like appearance, such as plant cells and *Blastocystis*, may be encountered when examining faeces, but these can fairly easily be distinguished from encysted amoebae. Air bubbles and fat globules may also be confused with cysts on casual examination. An amoebic cyst has a smooth outline and a definite thin cyst wall, and is highly refractile, especially in saline preparations. In addition, amoebic cysts in saline rarely show any inclusions such as nuclei, although refractile chromidial bars may be present in certain species.

Entamoeba histolytica (Fig. 1.2a, b)
The cysts are usually (though not invariably) spherical, and appear as circular bodies usually 10–15 μm in diameter. Cysts containing one, two or four nuclei may be found, and in formed stools the cysts will normally be quadrinucleate. The nuclei are rarely visible in saline preparations, but young cysts with one or two nuclei often contain one or more blunt chromidial bars which can be seen as refractile bodies. When the cyst is stained with iodine the chromidial bars cannot be seen, but nuclei usually show up well. The nuclear chromatin is often collected more thickly at one part of the nuclear membrane, giving a crescent-like appearance to the nucleus. Young cysts stained with iodine often show a diffuse brown-staining glycogen mass. The glycogen mass and chromidial bars have usually disappeared by the time the cyst is mature and quadrinucleate.

Entamoeba hartmanni
The cysts are similar to those of *E. histolytica* except that they are smaller, usually measuring 5–10 μm in diameter.

Entamoeba coli (Fig. 1.2c, d)
The cysts are usually spherical, appearing as circular bodies usually about 15–20 μm in diameter. They may contain up to eight nuclei, which are more easily seen in saline preparations than are the nuclei of *E. histolytica*. Chromidial bars may be seen in the young cysts, and these differ from those seen in cysts of *E. histolytica* in being faint and splinter-like, and often collected together into a bundle. When stained with iodine the cysts in formed stools usually show eight clearly stained nuclei that are seldom in the same focal plane and so can only be counted by altering the focus of the microscope. Young cysts, particularly those with two nuclei, show a densely stained dark brown glycogen mass. Chromidial bars are not visible in stained cysts.

Endolimax nana (Fig. 1.2e, f)
The cysts are spherical or ovoid, appearing as round or oval bodies about 6–10 μm in diameter. They are easily overlooked unless they are present in large numbers. Chromidial bars do not occur in the cysts, and the nuclei are not easily seen even after staining with iodine. Apart from the characteristic size and shape of the cysts, diagnosis depends on negative characteristics, the absence of obvious structures in the cysts.

Iodamoeba butschlii (Fig. 1.2g, h)
The cysts are variable in size, about 10–15 μm, and variable in shape, being spherical, ovoid or pointed at one end. In a freshly passed cyst the large glycogen mass is often visible as a clear space. The nucleus is not visible in saline preparations, and stains only faintly with iodine. Iodine-stained cysts show a densely stained dark brown glycogen mass, with a definite margin, occupying more than half the cysts.

Dientamoeba fragilis
The cyst is not known.

The Mastigophora

The class Mastigophora includes those protozoa that move actively by means of a flagellum (or several flagella) during all or part of their life. In addition, the body has a definite form, maintained by a firm pellicle on its outer surface. Some flagellates are devoid of a mouth opening, but some have an opening or 'cytosome' through which food is ingested. The species that parasitize man occur in various sites in the human body, notably in the blood, the tissues, the lumen of the gut, and the genital tract. The blood- and tissue-inhabiting species require an intermediate host to complete their life cycles, while the species occurring in the intestinal and genital tracts require only a single host, man. The intestinal flagellates pass directly from man to man, usually enclosed in a cyst but otherwise little altered. The vascular flagellates normally complete their life cycles in an insect host in which they undergo a fresh cycle of alteration and multiplication before they can again infect man. Most authorities believe that the cycle of flagellates in the insect vector differs from that of the malaria parasite in that there is no evidence of any sexual cycle.

Many flagellates inhabiting the gut of man may be found in the faeces, especially of dysentery cases in the tropics; others may be found in the mouth or genital tract. These parasites are nearly all harmless commensals; but two species, *Giardia intestinalis* and *Trichomonas vaginalis*, are associated with inflammatory lesions in heavy infections and for practical purposes may be regarded as pathogenic.

Giardia intestinalis

Giardia intestinalis (or *G. lambia*) has a world-wide distribution, especially in children under 10 years of age. Morphologically similar parasites are found in many vertebrates. The parasite lives in the small intestine, especially the duodenum, and perhaps in the gall bladder. It lies on top of the cells of the mucosa, attached by its sucker, and feeds on semidigested food of the host which is absorbed through the surface of the body. Division is by longitudinal fission. Multiplication is rapid, and pathogenic effects such as diarrhoea may occur in heavy infections. *Giardia* is normally discharged in the faeces in the form of cysts, but free flagellates are sometimes found. When in the faeces, the active forms may be seen 'skipping' up and down, but showing no progression. They may attach themselves to the slide or cover-slip, or to faecal fragments.

The cysts are produced in the lower part of the gut, in the terminal ileum and the colon. Encystment starts at the anterior end and proceeds backwards until a long oval cyst is produced, with uniform thick walls. The cysts cannot withstand desiccation, but will remain viable for about two weeks in moist faeces. Infection is by ingesting the mature cyst in contaminated food or water. The pathogenesis of *Giardia* is not well-defined. It may interfere with the absorption of fats, which can cause persistent diarrhoea with fatty stools. It is said to invade the gall bladder, causing cholecystitis and affecting the bile ducts. Diagnosis is by microscopical examination of faeces.

Trichomonas hominis

Trichomonas hominis has a world-wide distribution. It occurs in the large intestine, and is not pathogenic. It feeds on bacteria, starch and occasionally red blood cells.

Reproduction is by longitudinal fission, but this process is rarely seen. Cysts have not been described, and so the exact method of transmission is in some doubt. The active forms can survive at room temperature for at least two weeks, by rounding up and losing their flagella to produce a highly resistent form. Transmission may be by ingestion of either the active or the rounded resistant form.

Trichomonas tenax

Trichomonas tenax has a world-wide distribution, and is found in up to 26 per cent of diseased mouths and 11 per cent of healthy mouths. It is not pathogenic, and is rather similar to *T. hominis* in morphology and size.

Trichomonas vaginalis

Trichomonas vaginalis also has a world-wide distribution, and is found in both female and male urogenital tracts. It feeds on leucocytes and bacteria in the vaginal epithelium, and may cause inflammation of the vagina. It does not produce cysts, and transmission is often venereal. The pathogenic symptoms are apparently due to production of a substance which injures tissue cells.

Chilomastix mesnili

Chilomastix mesnili is another non-pathogenic parasite of the intestine of man. Its distribution is world-wide. It usually inhabits the large intestine, but may occur in the small intestine. Division of the trophozoites is by longitudinal fission, and transmission is by means of cysts. The cysts are pear-shaped or lemon-shaped, about 8 μm in diameter with the wall thickened at the anterior end.

Other flagellates

Not all intestinal flagellates are of medical importance. In addition to the non-pathogenic forms mentioned above, there are other non-pathogenic intestinal flagellates that may very rarely be found. These include species such as *Embadomonas intestinalis* and *Enteromonas hominis*. There is also a free-living species, *Bodo caudatus*, which is quite commonly found in stale stools or in urine vessels and may be mistaken for a parasite organism.

Medical aspects of giardiasis

Pathology

In light infections no changes in duodenal or jejunal morphology are found on biopsy. In heavier symptomatic infections partial villous atrophy and infiltration of the lamina propria with lymphocytes, plasma cells and poly-morphs is found on small-intestine biopsy. Conceivably the powerful sucking discs of trophozoites damage the microvilli of the small bowel mucosa. Actual mucosal invasion by the parasites is probably rare, but a mechanical barrier to the absorption of nutrient by numerous *Giardia* has been postulated. Immuno-logical reactions in the submucosa may lead to unusually rapid turnover of mucosal cells, with less mature cells at the villous tips producing reduced intestinal brush border enzymes. Bacterial colonization of the small bowel is found in heavy giardiasis infections and probably contributes to mucosal damage and the malabsorption found. As in bacterial gastroenteritis, giardiasis can be associated with diminished intestinal lactose secretion, causing diarrhoea and abdominal pain after ingestion of milk products.

Immunity and host resistance

Many human infections with *Giardia* are asymptomatic. In most, diarrhoea is short-lived (perhaps 4–14 days). The subject then becomes symptom-free but excretes cysts for some weeks. A minority of patients continue to have symptoms and excrete cysts for months or even years. It is not clear why some subjects have more chronic infections than others. The majority have no overt immunodeficiency, although giardiasis can be particularly chronic or severe when either humoral or cellular immune deficiencies are present. One attack of giardiasis does not protect against later infection.

In giardial infections IgG antibodies are found in the serum; lymphocytes and plasma cells in the intestinal wall initially produce IgM antibodies against *Giardia* and later IgG and IgA antibodies.

Clinical picture

The incubation period is commonly 1–3 weeks but may be much longer. Many of those infected do not have symptoms. Children are more likely to be sympto-matic than adults. Conditions such as immune deficiency, achlorhydria, previous gastrectomy and pancreatic disease predispose to giardiasis.

The onset is often acute with watery diarrhoea, abdominal cramps, fla-tulence, nausea, anorexia and abdominal distension. There may be mild systemic symptoms with low-grade fever, malaise and headaches. This acute phase often lasts for a few days to a week or two and is frequently diagnosed as bacterial gastroenteritis or travellers' diarrhoea. In most patients this completes the symptomatic phase, though they may continue to excrete cysts for months. In a minority, diarrhoea and abdominal discomfort continue intermittently for months or rarely for years. Malabsorption syndromes with malabsorption of fat, folic acid and D-xylose occur in the severely affected. Those with prolonged disease and malabsorption lose weight, become weak and anaemic, and produce three or four bulky foul-smelling stools daily with much flatus. Blood and mucus are not found in the stools. Abdominal discomfort, distension and 'gas' are often more prominent complaints than diarrhoea. Patients ethnically predisposed to lactase deficiency may suffer postgiardial lactase deficiency with diarrhoea and abdominal pain after milk products, even after successful elimination of the parasite. In children giardiasis may be associated with and contribute to protein–energy malnutrition.

Clinical diagnosis

Giardiasis should be considered in the differential diagnosis of acute, subacute and chronic diarrhoea (see Table 1.1), irritable bowel syndrome, peptic ulcer and gall bladder disease. It should always be sought as a possible, remediable cause of malabsorption. In assessing patients with chronic giardiasis, tests for malabsorption, blood folate levels, haemoglobin levels and red cell indices need evaluation. The possibility of immune deficiency should be thought about in severe, chronic giardiasis.

Treatment

The drug of choice is metronidazole (Flagyl). Two grams taken in one dose daily for 3 days is recommended for adults, and if necessary the tablets can be taken over the course of an hour. Alcohol should not be consumed when being treated with metronidazole as it may cause unpleasant 'Antabuse'-like reactions. Side effects are not usually severe with metronidazole but it may cause nausea, drowsiness, headache and skin rashes. The children's dosage is 7.5 mg/kg, 3 times daily for 7 days.

Alternatives are Tinidazole 2 g as a single dose for an adult; or mepacrine (Atebrine) 100 mg 3 times daily for 10 days for an adult. The latter may be used if metronidazole fails, but it can be toxic and in G-6-PD deficient subjects causes haemolysis.

Any nutritional deficiencies resulting from malabsorption will need correction. The possible adverse reactions to milk products have been mentioned. Giardiasis is often a family infection — other members should be screened and treated as necessary.

Medical aspects of trichomoniasis

Pathology

Trichomonas vaginalis can produce inflammatory changes on the mucosal surfaces of the vagina, urethra or occasionally the bladder. Probably 40 per cent of women and a high percentage of men harbouring the organism are asymptomatic. *Trichomonas vaginalis* may exist in the urethra, endocervical and urethral glands and prostate without inducing inflammation.

Symptoms

In women the symptoms are vaginal itching or burning, a yellowish and occasionally blood stained vaginal discharge and sometimes urinary frequency.

In men infection may cause urethritis.

Transmission

Transmission is by sexual intercourse, or by the sharing of toilet articles by women.

Treatment

Metronidazole 200 mg 3 time daily for 7 days, or 800 mg in the morning and 1.2 g at night for 2 days, is used. The sexual partner should be treated at the same time, and treatment repeated in 7 days.

Resistance to metronidazole has been reported, and Nimorazole in a single oral dose of 2 g can be used instead.

Laboratory indentification of intestinal and urogenital flagellates

These flagellates are identified by finding the active trophozoites, or sometimes the cysts, in the faeces, in discharges, or in smears from the mucous membranes. Trophozoites can normally be identified in fresh films, but if necessary their morphology can be confirmed in fixed, stained smears.

Giardia intestinalis

In diarrhoeic stools it is usual to find only the active trophozoites. The unencysted flagellate, which is found in a fresh film of faeces, has a characteristic appearance. It is a bilaterally symmetrical organism that looks rather like a pear from which a portion has been cut off obliquely from the anterior end (Fig. 1.3a). The flattened surface so formed is considered as the ventral surface. The body is 10–20 μm in length and tapers to a tail-like point which in the living animal is curved dorsally. The body is rigid, and the only changes of shape are due to the bending of the 'tail' and the altering contours of the 'sucker'. This sucker, or sucking disc, is a kidney-shaped depression on the ventral surface of the body, supported by two curved fibres. The animal attaches itself to the intestinal mucosa by means of this sucker. There are two nuclei and four pairs of flagella, but no mouth. The nuclei are oval vesicles that lie at the anterior end of the body, beneath the sucker and on either side of the median line. The nuclear membrane is thin and clear, and the karyosome is central and usually single. There are also two heavily staining rods, known as 'parabasal bodies', lying dorsal and transverse to the axostyles; but occasionally there may be only one, or even no parabasal body.

Cysts may be found in stools that may be loose or formed, and usually occur in large numbers. The cyst is ovoid in shape, about 10 μm in length and 8 μm in breadth. In unstained (saline) preparations of faeces, the cysts may show the axostyles, parts of the flagella and the margins of the sucking disc (or any of these structures). Such inclusions are diagnostic (Fig. 1.3b). Iodine-stained cysts show some or all of these inclusions, and may show nuclei at one end of the cyst. Newly formed cysts have two nuclei, but later the nuclei and the other internal structures are doubled, so that the mature cyst contains four nuclei.

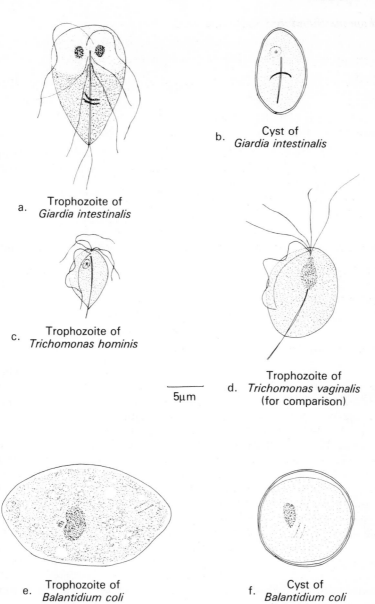

a. Trophozoite of
Giardia intestinalis

b. Cyst of
Giardia intestinalis

c. Trophozoite of
Trichomonas hominis

5μm

d. Trophozoite of
Trichomonas vaginalis
(for comparison)

e. Trophozoite of
Balantidium coli

f. Cyst of
Balantidium coli

20μm

Fig. 1.3 Intestinal Flagellates and Ciliates.

Trichomonas hominis

Cysts are not known, and the unencysted form is found in faeces. It is a small active body, ovoid or pear-shaped with a pointed caudal process, and between 5 μm and 14 μm in length (Fig. 1.3c). It is more plastic than *Giardia*, is more difficult to stain, and its characteristics are therefore not easily seen. The nucleus is a single oval vesicle and is anteriorly placed. The nuclear membrane is thin, and there is a small central karyosome. Anterior to the nucleus is a group of basal bodies from which arise three or four flagella that pass forwards, and one flagellum that passes backwards, running a spiral course to the posterior end of the body along the top of an undulating membrane. This last flagellum then continues as a posteriorly-trailing free flagellum. The base of the membrane is supported by a filament known as the 'basal fibre'. Through the centre of the body passes a skeletal rod which starts anteriorly, bends round the nucleus, runs posteriorly and finally protrudes outside the body as a pointed caudal process. At the anterior end of the body, by the side of the skeletal rod, is a slit-like mouth. The mouth is on the opposite side of the body to the undulating membrane.

Trichomonas tenax

This is generally similar morphologically to *T. hominis* and is almost the same size, but it differs from *T. hominis* in not possessing a posterior trailing free flagellum. The flagellate is found in scrapings from the teeth and gums, and occasionally from elsewhere in the oral cavity. Cysts are not known.

Trichomonas vaginalis

The unencysted flagellate is found in urine or in secretions from the vagina or prostate. *T. vaginalis* is easily confused with *T. hominis*, which may be present if the specimen is contaminated with faeces. *T. vaginalis* is the largest of the trichomonads found in man, being 7–23 μm long. Morphologically it is generally similar to *T. hominis*, but it is more spherical than the latter, the undulating membrane does not extend beyond two-thirds of the body length, and the marginal flagellum terminates at the postrior end of the membrane (Fig. 1.3d). The mouth is inconspicuous, and there is a well-developed parabasal body lying close to the nucleus. Cysts are not known.

Chilomastix mesnili

Both the encysted and unencysted forms may be found in the faeces. The unencysted flagellate is pear-shaped, with the posterior end drawn out into a pointed tail. It has a similar shape to *T. hominis* but is larger, being one of the largest intestinal flagellates in man. Its length is usually 10–15 μm, but it may be as long as 20 μm. The mouth is a large spiral longitudinal cleft in the anterior half of the body. The nucleus is an oval vesicle placed anteriorly. The basal bodies are placed near the anterior pole of the nucleus, six in a sphere, the three dorsal ones giving rise to three flagella which pass forwards as free flagella. The three ventral basal bodies give rise to two fibrils which support the lips, and to a flagellum in the depths of the mouth cleft which moves with a flickering motion and directs food particles into the mouth channel. There are no skeletal supports and no undulating membrane, and rigidity is given to the animal by the pellicle. The cytoplasm is vacuolated. The parasite moves in straight gliding movements.

The cyst is pear-shaped, about 8 μm in length, with the wall thickened at the pointed end. No internal structures are visible in the unstained cyst, but the stained cyst may show the nucleus (sometimes two nuclei), the fibrils supporting the mouth cleft, and perhaps a flagellum.

The Ciliophora

The members of this class are of various habits and morphology, but the general characteristics of all the ciliates parasitic in the intestine of mammals are similar. They are comparatively large, and have an abundant covering of cilia, which are extremely fine, short, hair-like organelles of locomotion. They have two nuclei, one somatic and one germinal, contractile excretory vacuoles, and a 'mouth'. In addition to reproduction by simple fission they undergo conjugation during which nuclear particles are exchanged. They pass from host to host as cyst. The only ciliate that is pathogenic to man is *Balantidium coli*, the cause of balantidial dysentery. It has a world-wide distribution, but is rare in man. It causes ulceration of the intestinal wall, and symptoms of colitis and diarrhoea.

Balantidium coli

B. coli occurs mainly in pigs, which are probably the natural host and in which the parasite is harmless, and is found also in monkeys and rats. The parasite exists in two stages, the trophozoite which is found in loose or dysenteric stools, and the encysted stage which is found in the stools of chronic cases and carriers.

The trophozoite is an oval body, about 70 μm long and 50 μm wide (Fig. 1.3e). There is a wide variation in size, but an infection is usually established with a race of homogenous size. In pigs the parasites are much larger, sometimes reaching 200 μm in length. The whole body is covered with cilia arranged in parallel, spiral rows. The anterior end is slightly more pointed than the posterior, and at the anterior end is a groove, the peristome, leading to a 'mouth', the cytostome, from which a funnel-shaped 'gullet', the cytopharynx, runs inwards for about one-third of the body length. There is no intestine. At the posterior end is a permanent 'anus', the cytopyge.

The cilia are short and of uniform size, except for those around the mouth which are stouter and longer. The shape of the body is normally constant, but the pellicle is not rigid and can be bent or distorted. The cytoplasm is divided into an outer thin layer of clear ectoplasm and a main mass of granular endoplasm. There are two nuclei, a large kidney-shaped macronucleus situated near the middle of the body and a small round micronucleus lying in the concavity of the macronucleus. There are two contractile vacuoles, one lying half-way up the body and one near the posterior end. They are connected by a narrow canal, and the posterior vacuole opens to the exterior by the anal pore. Food vacuoles circulate through the endoplasm, and contain particles such as starch, faecal fragments and erythrocytes.

Multiplication is by lateral transverse fission, often following a special mechanism of conjugation in which parts of the micronucleus are exchanged between individuals. Cysts are formed similarly to those of the intestinal amoebae. The trophozoite rounds off, discharges all food particles, and secretes a thick cyst wall. The cysts (Fig. 1.3h) are passed in the faeces, and may survive in moist conditions for several weeks. They are rapidly killed by desiccation. Infection is by swallowing the cysts as contaminants of food or drink, or by direct spread to the mouth by soiled hands.

Medical aspects of balantidiasis

Pathology

Perhaps less than 20 per cent of those infected have symptoms, but like *E. histolytica*, *B. coli* can invade the colonic mucosa causing necrosis and ulceration by virtue of its proteolytic secretions. As in invasive amoebiasis, secondary bacterial infection may occur and occasionally intestinal perforation. The ileum is occasionally involved but metastatic spread to the liver or elsewhere is rare.

Clinical picture and diagnosis

Invasive balantidiasis causes diarrhoea with the passage of blood and mucus, sometimes accompanied by fever, vomiting and wasting. Perforation is a potentially lethal complication.

The differential diagnosis is of the various forms of dysentery is listed in Table 1.1.

Treatment

Tetracycline 500 mg every 6 hours for 10 days is recommended. Paramomycin has also been used, but metronidazole is of uncertain value.

Laboratory diagnosis of balantidiasis

Trophozoites of *B. coli* are easily recognized by their size and morphology, there being no other similar parasites of man. Free-living ciliates are quite commonly found in specimens of faeces passed into unclean vessels; however, they are usually quite different morphologically from *Balantidium*, although the free-living *Paramoecium* is rather similar in appearance but is larger. When there is acute balantidial dysentery, the *Balantidium* can be differentiated from other ciliates by the presence of ingested erythrocytes.

The cysts are about 60 μm in diameter, spherical or ovoid, slightly yellowish or greenish in colour, and refractile. The cyst wall is thick, and the contained parasite frequently does not completely fill the cyst, leaving clear spaces at opposite sides of the cyst (Fig. 1.3f). In the young cyst the cilia are visible, but later they disappear. The macronucleus and the posterior contractile vacuoles are usually visible, although the vacuoles may have disappeared in the older cysts. Occasionally the parasite may divide within the cyst, so that two macronuclei are visible.

Prevention of intestinal protozoal infections

Infection of man is by the faecal-oral route, through direct contamination of foodstuffs — particularly vegetables growing at ground level — or indirect contamination of food by soiled fingers. Flies are important mechanical vectors of intestinal infections, the parasites being carried on their footpads. Animal reservoirs of infection are not important, except possibly in balantidiasis.

The most important preventive measures are general improvement in standards of hygiene and sanitation and in health education. A good supply of clean water facilitates washing of hands, food and utensils. Provision and proper use of latrines diminishes faecal contamination of food and the risk of infections being spread by flies. The most important measure in fly control is the proper disposal of refuse where flies might otherwise breed. Health education must include instruction about the use of latrines, hand washing after defaecation, protection of food from flies, and the concept of bacterial multiplication in food. Prevention of protozoal infection of food cannot be separated from prevention of bacterial infection of food.

Detection and treatment of asymptomatic cyst passers is not really practicable on a large scale, but it has some limited application; for example, food handlers in institutions should be periodically examined, and treated where possible. Mass treatment of populations is not feasible, and it has never been succcessfully carried out.

In many countries human faeces are often used as fertiliser, with consequent contamination of vegetables. Composting and storage of faeces before use usually destroy protozoal cysts and helminth eggs. Intestinal protozoal and helminth infections are often widespread within households, and if one infected individual is found then other members of the household should be examined and treated if necessary. Thorough washing of food, avoidance of the consumption of raw vegetables and fruit, protection of food from flies, and proper cooking of food are important. If water supplies are suspect, the water should be filtered and boiled if possible.

Further reading

Ackers JP, Knight R, Wright SG, Mendelson RM, Webster ADB, Ferguson A, *et al*. 1980 symposium on giardiasis. *Trans Roy Soc Tropical Med Hyg* 1980; **74**: 427–48.

Adams EB, MacLeod IN. Invasive amoebiasis: 1 Amoebic dysentery and its complications. *Medicine* 1977; **56**: 315–23.

Culbertson CG. Amoebic meningoencephalitis. In: Binford CH, Connor DH (eds) *Pathology of tropical and extraordinary diseases*. Tunbridge Wells: Castle House Publications, 1979, 317–24.

Juniper K. Amoebiasis. *Clin Gastroenterol* 1978; **7**: 3–29.

Knight R. Giardiasis, isosporiasis and balantidiasis. *Clin Gastroenterol* 1978; **7**: 31–47.

Meyer EA, Radulescu S. Giardia and giardiasis. *Adv Parasitol* 1979; **17**: 1–47.

Singh BN. *Pathogenic and non-pathogenic amoebae*. London: Macmillan 1975.

Wilmot AJ. *Clinical amoebiasis*. Oxford: Blackwell, 1962.

2

Sporozoa

All members of the class Sporozoa are parasitic, and they are characterized by a life-cycle which includes the production of spores. They do not have special organelles of locomotion such as cilia or flagella, except in the gametes, and have little capacity for movement during most of their life. They show 'alternation of generations', in which a single sexual generation is followed by a series of asexual generations. The sexual reproduction is known as gametogony, and results in the formation of gametes which fuse to form a zygote; the zygote then divides by sporogony to produce the infective spores. The asexual reproduction is known as schizogony, and during such reproduction the parasite multiplies by binary or multiple fission. There is often an 'alternation of hosts', with the asexual cycle in one host and the asexual cycle in another.

There is no generally accepted classification of the Sporozoa, but the sporozoan parasites of man are usually considered to be members of the two Orders Haemosporidia and Coccidia. These Orders are characterized by spores which contain numerous sporozoites and by mature trophozoites that are intracellular.

Malaria

The Order Haemosporidia includes the four species of parasites belonging to the genus *Plasmodium*, which produce malaria in man. The genus *Plasmodium* includes blood-inhabiting parasites in monkeys and other mammals, in birds, and in reptiles. Each host has its own appropriate species of parasite. Although transient infections have sometimes been transmitted experimentally from man to monkeys and from monkeys to man, there is no evidence that such transmission occurs in nature, so that animal reservoirs for human infections probably do not exist.

All plasmodia are closely adapted to parasitic life and have no free-living forms. All are transmitted in nature by their appropriate species of mosquitoes, in which invertebrate host the sexual cycle of the parasite occurs. The asexual cycle occurs in the vertebrate host, in the red blood cells, in the cells of the reticuloendothelial system and, in the earliest phases of the infection in man, in the parenchyma of the liver.

The sexual cycle of all the human plasmodia occurs only in, or rather is completed only in, the tissues of mosquitoes belonging to the genus *Anopheles* which have imbibed blood from patients with sexual forms (gametocytes) of *Plasmodium* in their peripheral blood. After multiplication in the insect, the parasites pass back to the human host mixed with the saliva of the biting insect.

The four species of *Plasmodium* which may give rise to malaria in man are *P. falciparum*, *P. vivax*, *P. malariae* and *P. ovale*. It is traditional to consider man as the definitive host in parasitic infections. However, some people now consider that in malaria the mammalian host is the intermediate host (because asexual reproduction occurs in this host) while the mosquito is the true definitive host (because sexual reproduction occurs in this host). Also for this reason, it is suggested that the parasite's association with the insect has been for longer than its association with man.

The complete life-cycle of the malaria parasite was not known until about the middle of this century, when the exoerythrocytic cycle in man was elucidated; and some details of the cycle are still not known. However, the life-cycles of the four malaria parasites of man are essentially similar, and as *P. falciparum* is probably the most important from the medical point of view, that species will be considered first.

Plasmodium falciparum

This parasite, the cause of malignant tertian malaria, occurs in many parts of the world, but essentially malignant tertian malaria is a disease of the tropics. This is probably because of the relatively high temperature required for its development in the mosquito vector. The development of *P. falciparum* is retarded below 18°C, and below 15°C the parasite will not be transmitted. Effective transmission of the infection really requires a sustained temperature of at least 20°C, and preferably one near 30°C.

It is convenient to start a consideration of the life-cycle (Fig. 2.1) at the stage when the infective form is injected into man by the feeding anopheline mosquito. The infective form, the sporozoite, is injected into the blood or lymph vessels or the subcutaneous tissue with the salivary secretion of the mosquito which is probing the tissue for its blood meal. The sporozoite is a thin, needle-like organism about 12 μm in length, with a central ovoid nucleus. It disappears from the blood within half an hour, and for about 8 days development proceeds outside the blood in the liver.

The development in the liver is known as 'pre-erythrocytic' development. About 2 days after the sporozoites disappear from the blood, parasites appear in the parenchymatous polyhedral cells of the liver as round bodies, about 8 μm in diameter, containing two or more nuclei. As the parasites grow the nuclei and the cytoplasm divide and the parasite becomes progressively larger, pushing aside the nucleus of the liver cell, and distending the liver cell until by about 5–7 days later the liver cell has become a lobulated ovoid mass, some 60 μm in diameter, containing about 40 000 merozoites. No pigment is produced in the liver schizont. About 8 days after the inoculation of the parasite as a sporozoite, the merozoites are liberated from the schizont into the blood and develop to become the asexual forms, the trophozoites.

The young trophozoite is a small vesicular body, about 1 μm in diameter, which in stained blood films appears as a small fine ring of cytoplasm with the chromatin in one or two small dots or as a longer bar (Fig. 2.2). It feeds on the parasitized erythrocyte, enlarges until it is about half the size of the erythrocyte, and becomes more solid. At this stage of development the erythrocytes infected with *P. falciparum* tend to clump together, and these clumps of infected cells are trapped in the small capillaries of the internal organs. The nucleus of the mature trophozoite then divides, and with it the cytoplasm, until the parasite (now a

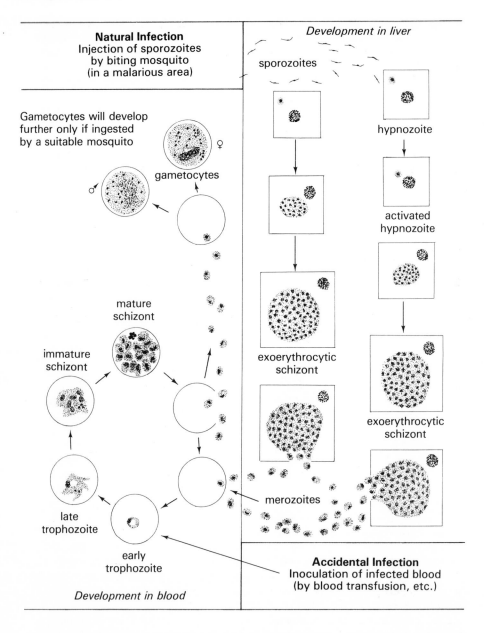

Fig. 2.1   The Life Cycle of Malaria in Man. Sporozoites injected by a female *Anopheles* mosquito circulate in the blood for a short time before penetrating the liver parenchyma cells, where they develop into exoerythrocytic schizonts. Some of the sporozoites of *Plasmodium vivax* (and probably of *P. ovale*) will lie dormant in the liver as hypnozoites which will later cause relapses. Hypnozoites do not occur in infections with *P. falciparum* and *P. malariae*; persistence of these two infections occurs only in the blood, so there are recrudescences but not true relapses.

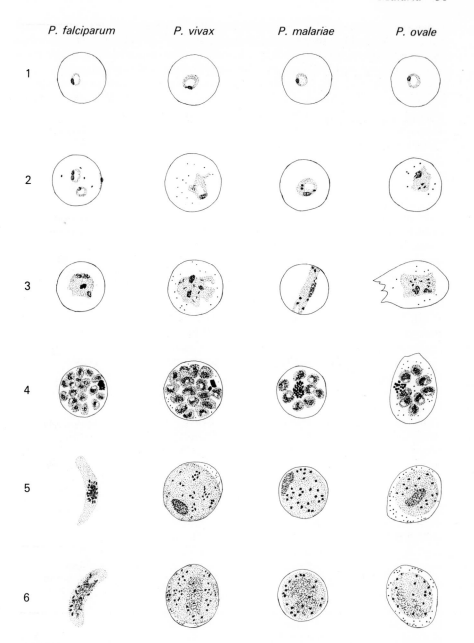

Fig. 2.2 Erythrocytic stages of Malaria in Man.
1. Early trophozoites or 'rings'; 2. Late trophozoites; 3. Late trophozoites and pre-schizonts; 4. Mature schizonts; 5. Female gametocytes; 6. Male gametocytes.

schizont) contains between 6 and 24 (usually 12–16) merozoites. These merozoites are 1 μm in diameter, and arranged around an aggregation of residual cytoplasm and pigment (Fig. 2.2). The red cell then ruptures in the static backwaters of the visceral circulation, liberating the merozoites which invade neighbouring red blood cells. The pigment is taken up by the leucocytes, mononuclear phagocytes and endothelial cells. The newly infected red blood cells are then washed out into the peripheral circulation. This cycle of development takes 2 days, but in the early stages of an infection the cycles may not all be synchronous. In established infections, rupture of the infected erythrocytes, and therefore the fever, occurs regularly on the third day — hence the name 'tertian malaria'.

Later the early sexual forms, the gametocytes, are produced. Ten to fourteen days after the onset of the clinical infection, the gametocytes (Fig. 2.2) appear fully grown in the peripheral blood. Unlike the formation of schizonts, the process of formation of gametocytes cannot be reproduced in culture, so less is known of its course. The gametocytes undergo no further development in man; instead, they remain circulating in the blood until they either perish (normally after 30–60 days, but they may live longer) or are ingested by a blood-sucking insect. If the insect happens to be an anopheline mosquito, the next phase of the life-cycle begins.

When the mosquito takes a blood meal, any malaria parasites in the blood are sucked up with the blood into its mid-gut (Fig. 2.1). Any asexual forms which are present in the blood perish rapidly, but sexual forms begin to develop in the mosquito's stomach as the temperature of the blood falls. First the male and female gametocytes rapidly lose their crescent form and round up, escaping from the remnants of their enclosing red blood cells. Development is different in the male and female gametocytes. In the male the nucleus divides, and four to eight long cytoplasmic processes project from the surface, each containing a small cylinder of nuclear chromatin. Ten minutes after the ingestion of the blood-meal these processes break off to form microgametes which swim in the fluid blood. This process is known as exflagellation. The original mass of the gametocyte from which the microgametes have originated then disintegrates. In the female gametocyte the nucleus divides and part of the nuclear material is extruded as what are usually referred to as polar bodies (although it has recently been suggested that the division of the gametocytes is not a reduction division, so that the extruded nuclear particles cannot be polar bodies). The cell has now become the uninuclear macrogamete, and is pierced by a microgamete to form the zygote. The zygote becomes amoeboid, elongates until it is about 20 μm × 3 μm, and forms the actively motile ookinete.

The ookinete then bores into the wall of the mosquito's stomach and rounds off to form an oocyst under the structureless outer layer of the gut wall. The oocyst becomes divided into a numbers of sporoblasts, which divide by longitudinal fission to form large number of sporozoites, each about 12 μm long. This whole cycle of development takes 8–20 days, depending on the temperature. The oocyst then bursts, releasing the sporozoites into the haemocoele of the mosquito, and they become generally distributed throughout the organs of the fly, in the legs, palps and elsewhere. Most of the sporozoites make their way, or are carried, to the salivary glands. Finally they come to lie free in the saliva, with which they are discharged when the insect is probing before taking a blood meal. The mosquito may take numerous blood meals during the remainder of its life, discharging sporozoites the whole time.

Plasmodium vivax

P. vivax is more widespread than *P. falciparum*, and occurs in temperate regions as well as in the tropics and subtropics. This is probably because it can develop in the mosquito at a lower temperature than can *P. falciparum*. It is the cause of 'benign tertian' malaria, which is rarely fatal in uncomplicated cases.

Apart from a few minor differences, the life-cycle and the morphology of the stages of the parasite in the mosquito are identical with those of *P. falciparum*. There are, however, important differences in the part of the life-cycle that occurs in man, the main difference being that *P. vivax* undergoes its entire asexual cycle in the peripheral blood as well as in the internal blood vessels. Infection occurs when sporozoites are injected into the tissues by the feeding mosquito, and the pre-erythrocytic development takes place in the parenchymal cells of the liver. About 4 days after infection schizonts can be seen in the liver, and the schizonts reach maturity about 7 days afterwards. The mature schizont is about 40 μm in diameter, completely fills the liver cell, and contains at least 10 000 merozoites. The schizont then ruptures, and the released merozoites enter the red blood cells to initiate the asexual erythrocytic cycle.

Some of the sporozoites, however, remain dormant in the liver as 'hypnozoites', and these may develop into tissue schizonts some time later. These delayed tissue schizonts are the cause of the relapses associated with benign tertian malaria. Hypnozoites probably occur also in infections with *P. ovale*, but they do not occur in infections with *P. falciparum* or *P. malariae*. Persistence of these two infections occurs only in the blood, so there are recrudescences but not relapses.

The cycle in the blood is essentially the same as that of *P. falciparum*, but all stages occur in the peripheral circulation (Fig. 2.2). The mature trophozoite divides to produce a schizont containing 12–24 (average 16) merozoites, each about twice the size of the merozoites of *P. falciparum*. The whole cycle takes about 48 hours. The gametocytes appear a little earlier than in *P. falciparum*, usually within 8 days of the onset of the erythrocytic cycle.

The two remaining species of malaria parasites, *P. malariae* and *P. ovale*, have a similar erythrocytic cycle to *P. vivax*, although *P. malariae* requires a longer period (72 hours) to complete its asexual cycle and also a longer period for its development in the mosquito. This longer period results in a smaller proportion of mosquitoes surviving to the stage at which they become infective, so that there is a tendency for *P. malariae* to die out where anopheline mosquitoes are few in number. This tendency is to some extent compensated for by the fact that *P. malariae* persists in the human host for longer periods than do the other species.

Plasmodium malariae

This parasite has a world-wide but localized distribution, and is the cause of quartan malaria. Development in the liver is slower than in *P. falciparum*, but there are no hypnozoites. The full asexual cycle in the blood takes 72 hours, as compared with 48 hours for the other species, and after this period the mature schizont contains 8–12 merozoites (Fig. 2.2).

Plasmodium ovale

This is another tertian parasite, and it is the rarest of the human plasmodia. It it found in all continents except Europe. Its erythrocytic cycle resembles that of *P. vivax* in that it occupies 48 hours and takes place in the general circulation. Hypnozoites probably occur. The morphology of the erythrocytic stages is intermediate between those of *P. malariae* and *P. vivax* (Fig. 2.2).

Pathogenesis of malaria

This account will mainly concern *falciparum* malaria, the most serious form of the disease. The pathogenic effects of malaria are related to the erythrocytic stage of the parasite. The pre-erythrocytic hepatic stages and the gametocytes cause no significant damage.

Changes in the blood

Rupture of red blood cells on the emergence of malarial merozoites causes release of red blood cell constituents and malarial waste products into the circulation. These are pyrogenic, causing fever. In primary attacks the fever is irregular and sustained for some days. Later, erythrocytic schizogony becomes synchronized and fever tends to recur at 48-hour intervals; sometimes rather less than 48 hours, hence the term 'malignant subtertian' malaria. The tertian fever refers to fever every third day.

Anaemia occurs when red cell destruction exceeds production, and during febrile attacks there is some inhibition of marrow erythropoietic production. The anaemia is normocytic, and indirect bilirubin is increased in the blood. Unparasitized as well as parasitized cells are haemolysed by complement-mediated immune reactions when malaria antigen coats uninfected red cells. The direct Coombs test is sometimes positive. Occasionally there is massive intravascular haemolysis with saturation of haptoglobulins, haemoglobinaemia and haemoglobinuria — 'malarial haemoglobinuria' (Blackwater fever). The cause of this is unclear, but it has been associated with states of incomplete immunity, irregular drug prophylaxis, and sometimes with the use of quinine which itself can cause haemolysis. Malarial haemoglobinuria can result in severe anaemia, shock and renal failure.

Other changes in the blood include thrombocytopenia and leucopenia, mainly due to reduction in polymorphonuclear cells. Sometimes there is a monocytosis. Evidence of consumption coagulopathy may be present, but there are doubts regarding its significance in pathogenesis. Hypoglycaemia has recently been recorded and may be of significance in cerebral malaria.

Circulatory changes

Obstruction of capillaries occurs in *falciparum* malaria, and this results in anoxic damage to various organs including the brain, kidneys, liver, lungs and gastrointestinal tract. This contributes to the causation of cerebral malaria, renal and hepatic failure, and the diarrhoea found in patients with malaria. Various mechanisms are thought to cause capillary obstruction; these include adherence of parasitized red cells to capillary walls, and damage to capillary epithelium (possibly mediated by kinin liberation) with leakage of plasma into the tissues and resultant local haemoconcentration and sludging of blood. In pulmonary capillaries damage may result in pulmonary oedema.

There are other changes in the general circulation. There is peripheral vasoconstriction in the initial 'cold' stage of the febrile paroxysm, followed by vasodilation in the hot stage with diminished effective plasma volume and postural hypotension. Vasoconstriction has been demonstrated experimentally in some visceral arteries in animals, and may contribute to hepatic and renal damage.

Immunologically mediated changes

Hyperplasia of elements of the reticuloendothelial system contributes to splenic enlargement. Immune complexes in glomeruli lead to temporary nephritic changes in acute *falciparum* malaria and sometimes cause permanent progressive nephritis in *malariae* malaria. Immune mediated haemolysis has already been mentioned.

Suppression of host immunity is induced by acute *falciparum* malaria in children, resulting in increased susceptibility to other infections and reduced responses to immunization. Burkitt's lymphoma may be initiated by malarial-induced suppression of the normal immune response to Epstein–Barr virus.

Nutritional effects

Infections have a considerable influence in precipitating malnutrition in children on marginal diets. In malaria an increased metabolic rate, production of immunoglobulins, red cell destruction, anorexia, vomiting and a temporary malabsorption state during acute attacks all predispose to malnutrition.

Other suggested pathogenic mechanisms in malaria include the effects of endotoxin release and a toxic depression of cellular mitochondrial function.

Vivax and *ovale* malaria

In *vivax* malaria the extent of red cell invasion is limited, and rarely more than 2 per cent of red cells are parasitized. Serious complications occur uncommonly, although splenic rupture with fatal consequences has been recorded after minimal trauma or even spontaneously. Fatalities are uncommon, but rarely the very old, very young and very frail may succumb. The effects of *ovale* malaria are similar to those found in *vivax* malaria.

Malariae malaria

Malariae infections are usually not fatal because invasion of the red cells is restricted to about 1 per cent. It has been suggested that *P. vivax* invades only young cells and *P. malariae* attacks only old cells. Nevertheless the parasite is an important cause of nephrotic syndrome in children, and is remarkably persistent.

Immunity and host resistance in malaria

Immunity is slowly acquired through repeated malarial infections and diminishes if the host ceases to be exposed to malarial infection for some years. Malarial immunity is species specific, and to an extent is specific for different geographical strains of the parasite. Newborn infants of immune mothers have resistance to malaria because of transplacental transfer of antimalarial immunoglobulin G. This passive immunity wanes and the child becomes susceptible to malaria after about four months. In an area of heavy and continuous malarial transmission (a holoendemic situation) children usually gain substantial immunity by the age of 5 or 6 years.

Both T lymphocytes and B lymphocytes are involved in malarial immunity. The intracellular position of the parasite may protect it from immune processes, but the existence of antibodies penetrating and acting within the red cell has been postulated. Merozoites are susceptible to immune attack while in the plasma.

Hepatic stages of the parasite escape immune attack. It is suspected that malarial parasites may undergo antigenic variation as a variety of immune evasion.

It is now possible to culture *P. falciparum* parasites *in vitro*, and investigations are proceeding in attempts to produce effective malaria vaccines.

Diminished susceptibility to malaria

Some individuals are less susceptible than others to malarial infection and its effects. Heterozygote sicklers (AS) are less likely to die of malaria in childhood than those with normal haemoglobin. Haemoglobin S may be less favourable to parasite growth; infection of the red cell induces sickling and speedy removal of the infected cell from the circulation by the reticuloendothelial system. The increased survival rate of heterozygous sicklers explains the persistence of the deleterious S gene in malarious areas (balanced polymorphism).

Haemoglobin F may be less favourable for malarial metabolism than haemoglobin A; this could give some protection to newborns and in thalassaemia minor. Glucose-6-phosphate-dehydrogenase (G-6-P-D) deficiency also appears to provide some protection against malaria. The presence of the Duffy blood group antigen on the red cell surface is necessary for the attachment and invasion of *P. vivax*; there is a very low prevalence of the Duffy antigen in West Africans, and *P vivax* infection hardly ever occurs in them.

Increased susceptibility to malaria

Pregnancy causes diminished immunity to malaria, especially in primigravidae. Splenectomy increases susceptibility to malaria in those previously immune.

Epidemiology of malaria

Malaria has differing epidemiological features in various endemic areas, largely depending on the intensity and continuity of malarial transmission. The classical extreme situations are known as stable and unstable malaria, and the characters of these are given in Table 2.1.

Table 2.1 Classical characteristics of malaria

	Stable malaria	Unstable malaria
Transmission	Continuous and often intense	Discontinuous, often seasonal, and maximal in the rainy season
Immunity	Usually good over the age of 5 years	Usually poor in community
Severe malaria occurs	Mainly in children	At all ages
Splenomegaly	High prevalence (over 50%) in children aged 2–9; low incidence in adults	May be present in all age groups
Epidemics	Do not occur	Do occur, and the mortality rate may be high

The degree of transmission depends on, among other factors, the numbers of anopheline mosquitoes present and their efficiency as vectors. The mosquito population is affected by climatic factors such as high or low temperatures, humidity, and the availability of breeding places. The West African coast is an example of a stable malaria area; malaria is unstable in some Indian highland areas.

Clinical features of malaria

Falciparum malaria

Primary attacks of *falciparum* malaria in non-immunes may cause serious illness with a high mortality rate unless treated. Once immunity has been acquired, sporadic but comparatively mild attacks of malaria occur.

Incubation period
This is usually 10–14 days, but maybe only a few days or may be prolonged for weeks or months if prophylactics have been taken. In the UK clinical *falciparum* malaria usually develops with a month of return from malarious areas, but in 5–10 per cent of cases it occurs later than this.

Onset
This is often abrupt with high fever, but sometimes insidious with prodromal

symptoms of malaise, headache, anorexia and muscular pains before parasites are detectable in the blood.

Evolution
For the first week there is a severe systemic febrile illness with irregular fever, headache, body pains, postural hypotension and often vomiting. Deterioration with the onset of complications can appear at any time. The patient becomes weakened and anaemic, and the temperature chart may begin to show the typical tertian or subtertian rhythm with bouts of fever lasting 8–12 hours every 48 hours or so. Classically the fever (ague) fits pass through cold, hot and sweating stages.

Clinical signs include anaemia, mild jaundice and tender hepatosplenomegaly. Enlargement of the spleen takes several days to appear in a primary attack.

Treatment should cause rapid improvement unless the illness is very advanced. Even without treatment many patients avoid complications, and illness gradually subsides as the patient gains immunity.

Recrudescence is not uncommon but does not usually occur after one year.

Complicated malaria

Complications of malaria cause serious morbidity and mortality.

Cerebral malaria
This is a serious acute encephalopathy. Mental confusion and severe headache proceed to stupor, coma, hyperthermia and death unless treated. There may be generalized convulsions, particularly in children, and occasionally focal signs such as hemiplegia. Evolution may be fulminant, the patient dying within a few hours — so treatment is very urgent. The CSF may be under increased pressure but its composition is usually normal and cell-free. Pathologically the brain shows petechial haemorrhages, congestion and sometimes oedema; microscopically cerebral capillaries are blocked by parasitized erythrocytes and some are surrounded by ring haemorrhages. Investigations in Thailand using computerized tomography have shown that the brain is not usually swollen with increased intracranial pressure in cerebral malaria.

Gastrointestinal malaria
Vomiting is common in malaria, and sometimes there is severe diarrhoea (choleraic or dysenteric malaria) due to damage to the intestinal epithelium. Hepatogenous jaundice with centrilobular necrosis may occur, and occasionally hepatocellular failure.

Acute renal failure
This is not rare and results from circulatory changes, systemic hypotension and renal cortical vasoconstriction, which lead to tubular necrosis. Oliguria is a warning sign. Haemodialysis or peritoneal dialysis may be required.

Algid malaria
This is a serious shock syndrome, the precise cause of which is not clear. Con-

sumption coagulopathy and increased capillary permeability with diminished vascular volume and Gram-negative septicaemia may all be factors.

Pulmonary oedema
This is uncommon in severe form, but frequently fatal. There is increasing dyspnoea, cough, and expectoration of frothy and blood-stained sputum. Crepitations are heard on chest auscultation.

Malaria in children
In holoendemic areas malaria is most prevalent in children. Infants show refusal to feed, vomiting, diarrhoea, cough and febrile convulsions. After repeated attacks there is wasting, failure to thrive, marked hepatosplenomegaly and anaemia. Children are particularly liable to cerebral malaria, hyperthermia, anaemia and shock. In some localities 10 per cent of children may die of malaria before the age of 5 years. Malaria is often associated with intercurrent infections and malnutrition.

Malaria in pregnancy
Diminution of maternal immunity in pregnancy (especially the first) can lead to febrile attacks and anaemia. Abortion, stillbirth or premature labour are complications. Infection of the placenta is associated with the birth of small babies that have a higher mortality rate than those of normal weight in the first weeks of life. Congenital infection is rare in infants of immune mothers, but is occasionally seen in children of nonimmunes.

Transfusion malaria
Malaria can be transmitted by blood transfusion, sometimes years after the donor has left malarious areas; indeed, the parasites of *P. malariae* may persist in the blood for over 10 years. Transfusion malaria can be a puzzling cause of fever after transfusion, particularly if it develops following an operation.

In highly malarious areas it is impracticable to reject blood from possibly malarious individuals, and it is not generally practicable to treat the donor before donation. It is often preferable to give the recipient a course of anti-malaria drugs during and after the transfusion. Transfusion malaria does not have an exoerythrocytic stage, so treatment with primaquine is unnecessary even if the infections are with *vivax* or *ovale*. Blood that has been stored for more than 10 days is safe.

In non-malarious areas people with a history of malaria are not usually acceptable as donors. However, people who have resided in malarious areas may if necessary be screened by the IFA test.

Malaria has also been transmitted between drug addicts who hand on contaminated syringes for injecting themselves.

Vivax and ovale malaria

The incubation period of *vivax* malaria ranges from 10 days to 8 months or longer. The general clinical features are similar to those of *falciparum* malaria but are less serious, and complicated malaria as described above is not a feature. Occasional fatalities are found in debilitated subjects and from ruptured spleens. Relapses due to hypnozoites usually occur up to 2 years after infection, but they can occur up to 5 years later. *Ovale* malaria is clinically similar to *vivax* malaria.

Malariae malaria

This is less common than *falciparum* or *vivax* malaria but can cause quite severe disease, in particular an immune complex nephritis causing a nephrotic syndrome in children which usually progresses to renal failure. The incubation period is longer than for other varieties (18 days to several weeks) and the disease may recrudesce for 20–40 years, presumably owing to a persistent low-grade parasitaemia.

Tropical splenomegaly

Some individuals living in malarious areas develop progressive and eventually massive splenomegaly. No other cause apart from malaria can be identified in these cases, and it is considered to be an abnormal immune response to malarial infection. It is possibly due to ineffective T-cell control of B-cell immuno-globulin production. These patients have high levels of malarial antibody and IgM. Pathologically the spleen is congested and shows evidence of infarcted areas and fibrosis, often with adhesions to parietal peritoneum and diaphragm. The liver is enlarged, the sinusoids being infiltrated with lymphocytes and plasma cells; the Kuppfer cells are increased in number.

Clinically the patient complains of pain in the splenic area and weakness. He or she has splenomegaly, moderate hepatomegaly, anaemia with a haemoglobin of 6–8 g/dl, evidence of hypersplenism with leucopenia and thrombocytopenia, and the immunoglobin changes noted above. These patients remain chronically ill. The diagnosis depends on excluding other causes for splenomegaly, the blood changes already decribed and, if necessary, liver biopsy.

If antimalarials are given on a long-term basis as for malaria prophylaxis (chloroquine 300 mg base weekly, proguanil 100 mg daily) the spleen will gradually shrink after several months, and the anaemia will improve. Anti-malarials should be continued permanently if possible. Splenectomy is not advisable; the operation is technically difficult and the long-term prognosis is poor after splenectomy.

Clinical diagnosis of malaria

Malaria cannot be distinguished from other febrile illnesses on clinical grounds or supposed therapeutic response; parasitological diagnosis is needed. Tender-ness over the splenic area and later splenomegaly, anaemia and characteristic fever patterns support the diagnosis. Some of the differential diagnoses of malaria are shown in Table 2.2.

Blood changes

Haemolytic anaemia of varying degree follows an attack of malaria. Reticulo-cytosis occurs after about a week, or following therapy. Moderate leucopenia

Table 2.2 Some differential diagnoses of malaria

Clinical syndrome	Differential diagnosis	Comments
Systemic febrile illness	Influenza	Commonest misdiagnosis in the UK; patients usually have respiratory symptoms
	Typhoid	Abdominal discomfort and tenderness
	Arbovirus infection	May have rash and lymphadenopathy
	Amoebic liver abscess	Tender enlarged liver; polymorphonuclear leucocytosis
	Relpasing fever	Clinically similar to malaria
	Visceral leishmaniasis	Massive splenomegaly
Fever and jaundice	Viral hepatitis	Bilirubinuria present
	Yellow fever	Haemorrhagic signs prominent
Fever, diarrhoea and vomiting in children	Gastroenteritis	Suspect malaria in children with high temperatures and diarrhoea
Cerebral signs of acute encephalopathy	Pyogenic meningitis Viral encephalitis	Early diagnosis vital; lumbar puncture often essential for diagnosis
	Febrile convulsions	
Fever and pulmonary oedema	Severe pneumonia	Sputum probably purulent in pneumonia
Tropical splenomegaly	Chronic myeloid leukaemia Visceral leishmaniasis Portal hypertension	Blood and marrow examination needed

and thrombocytopenia are often found in *falciparum* malaria. Numerous biochemical changes may be present, including elevated indirect and direct bilirubin, transaminases, serum potassium and blood urea. Serum albumin, sodium and glucose may be lowered.

Management of *falciparum* malaria

The objectives are to eliminate the parasites, correct any physiological abnormality and relieve symptoms. It is important to monitor progress to detect complications early and to ensure that the given chemotherapy is effective. Management is therefore specific, supportive, symptomatic and supervisory.

Specific treatment

4-aminoquinolines such as chloroquine and amodiaquine are the most rapid and efficient means of destroying erythrocytic parasites. Chloroquine acts by combining with the parasites' DNA and preventing passage of genetic material and by interfering with parasite nutrition. The drugs act on the dividing stages and are therefore known as schizontocides. Unfortunately there is widespread chloroquine resistance in South East Asia, Eastern India, Central and South American and East and Central Africa. There are different grades of resistance: in R1 resistance the asexual parasites disappear in 7 days but there is subsequent recrudescence; in R2 resistance parasites are reduced but do not disappear; and in R3 resistance there is no marked reduction in parasitaemia.

Dosage schedules for 4-aminoquinolines
Oral therapy is used whenever possible, except for seriously ill patients and those who cannot retain the drug because of vomiting.

The oral dose for adults is chloroquine base 600 mg (4 tablets) initially, followed by 300 mg in 6 hours and 300 mg daily for 3 days. The children's dosage is 10 mg/kg base initially, followed by 5 mg/kg base in 6 hours and 5 mg/kg base daily for 3 days.

Amodiaquine is given in an adult dose of 600 mg initially followed by 400 mg daily for 3 days. Semi-immune subjects will respond to smaller doses of 4-aminoquinolines, e.g. 600 mg base for an adult in a single dose, but in areas of emerging chloroquine resistance the full dose should be given.

If parenteral use is clearly indicated, chloroquine sulphate should be given slowly in a drip — 5 mg/kg with a maximum dose of 300 mg in 250 ml saline over 4 hours. This can be repeated in 8 hours, and oral therapy begun as soon as possible.

Intramuscular chloroquine is less satisfactory but can be used in the same dosage as for intravenous use. The dose of 5 mg/kg *must not be exceeded* in children, as death from cardiorespiratory arrest and convulsions may follow overdosage with parenteral chloroquine. Parenteral quinine (see below) given intravenously is preferable to parenteral chloroquine in complicated malaria.

Toxicity of 4-aminoquinolines
Abdominal discomfort, vomiting, headache and dizziness may follow oral

dosage. A severe generalized pruritus is common in dark-skinned people and is probably partly an allergic phenomenon.

Prolonged use over years with a total dose of 100 g or more has led to irreversible retinal degenerative changes.

Cardiorespiratory depression after parenteral use has been mentioned above.

Chloroquine-resistant malaria

If there is likelihood of a chloroquine-resistant strain being present, other drugs must be used. Quinine is a rapidly acting schizontocide, probably acting by interfering with DNA replication.

For an adult with uncomplicated malaria, quinine sulphate 650 mg 3 times daily is given orally for 5 days, after which 1.5 g (3 tablets) of Fansidar is given. Fansidar contains sulfadoxine and pyrimethamine, and interferes with the parasites' folate metabolism. There is some resistance to quinine in Thailand, and resistance to Fansider in Thailand and Kenya.

New drugs that may be used in such situations (if available) include mefloquine in a single dose of 1 g, and qinghaosu (Artemosine). When Fansidar resistance is suspected, quinine may be used combined with tetracycline 250 mg 6-hourly for 10 days. Toxic effects of quinine, known as cinchonism, include tinnitus, headache, nausea, abdominal pain and visual disturbances.

Intravenous quinine dihydrochloride is probably the best parenteral drug for cerebral and severe malaria. It should be given slowly in doses of 10 mg/kg in 10 ml/kg of saline or 5% dextrose over 4 hours. Workers in Thailand have used a loading dose of 20 mg/kg in areas where the parasite is relatively resistant to quinine. The initial dose may be repeated 12-hourly until oral therapy can be started.

Intravenous quinine can cause hypotensive shock and the patient needs careful monitoring.

Supportive treatment

Measures to correct physiological upsets may be needed, including transfusion for significant anaemia (PCV under 20 per cent) and treatment of renal failure. Care must be taken not to overload the circulation with saline as this may cause pulmonary or cerebral oedema. Intravenous frusemide and oxygen are given for pulmonary oedema, and in desperate cases positive-pressure-assisted respiration and venesection have been used.

Prolonged haemolysis may induce folate deficiency; if so, folic acid is given. Corticosteroids are no longer recommended for cerebral malaria.

Other problems encountered include (1) convulsions, (2) aspiration pneumonia, (3) hyperpyrexia, (4) hypoglycaemia, (5) shock, (6) Gram-negative septicaemia, and (7) renal failure. Appropriate preventive and therapeutic measures include (1) anticonvulsants, (2) correct positioning (semiprone) of comatose patients, and antibiotics, (3) cool sponging if temperature rises above 38.5°C, (4) blood sugar monitoring in patients with disturbed consciousness, and intravenous glucose if necessary, (5) correction of hypovolaemia, treatment of bacterial infections and possibly intravenous dopamine, (6) large doses of crystalline penicillin and gentamycin or tobramycin for septicaemia, and (7) monitored fluid replacement with normal saline, intravenous frusemide and peritoneal dialysis or haemodialysis for renal failure.

Symptomatic treatment

Simple analgesics such as paracetamol suffice for headaches and body aches in most cases. Sedation may be needed for restlessness, and anticonvulsants may be necessary.

Supervisory management

Careful monitoring of non-immune patients with malaria is necessary. Input and output charts, blood urea and haemoglobin levels, and liver function tests are needed. Daily blood films for parasites are desirable in the early stages to ensure that the infection is responding.

Malaria is a relatively mild illness in semi-immunes and is often treated on an outpatient basis.

Treatment of *vivax, ovale* and *malariae* malaria

For *vivax* and *ovale* parasites, the acute attack is treated with chloroquine as for *falciparum* malaria. Chloroquine resistance has not been found in these parasites. Relapses are prevented by using primaquine which acts on hypnozoites in the liver. Following the chloroquine, 15 mg of primaquine is given daily (in 1 or 2 doses) for 2 weeks. Some strains of *vivax* (e.g. from New Guinea) may need larger doses — 30 mg daily for 2 weeks. Primaquine may cause haemolysis in those with G-6-P-D deficiency, and potential recipients of primaquine should be screened for this abnormolity before treatment. Those deficient may usually be safely treated with 45 mg primaquine once weekly for 6 weeks.

Malariae malaria responds to treatment with chloroquine.

Individual prophylaxis of malaria

This has become a difficult problem because of the extent and varying degrees of chloroquine resistance, and the occasional serious toxic effects of Fansidar and Maloprim (dapsone 100 mg and pyrimethamine 12.5 mg in each tablet).

Prophylaxis is advised for non-immune visitors to malarious areas; in some cases in endemic areas for local children under the age of 5 years; for pregnant women; and temporarily for local people returning to infected areas after long residence in Europe.

Chloroquine or amodiaquine are excellent prophylactics in areas where the parasites are chloroquine sensitive. They are taken in doses of 300 mg base (2 tablets) or 400 mg base (2 tablets) weekly respectively.

When chloroquine resistance is suspected, Fansidar 1 tablet or Maloprim 1 tablet and chloroquine 300 mg base are taken weekly. Chloroquine is a better prophylactic against *vivax* malaria than the others, and the parasite is always sensitive to it. Prolonged continuous use of chloroquine prophylaxis for over 3 years is not advised because of dangers of retinopathy. There is widespread malaria resistance to pyrimethamine (Daraprim) used alone, and also to pro-guanil (Paludrine), although the latter may still be effective in many areas in a dose of 200 mg daily.

Fansidar and Maloprim prophylaxis has been associated with agranulocytosis in a few cases (perhaps 1/2000 in the case of 2 Maloprim tablets a week). Agranulocytosis is rare when 1 Maloprim tablet weekly is given for prophylaxis.

Malaria prophylaxis considerably reduces the chance of infection, but cannot be absolutely guaranteed to prevent malaria. Whenever used it should be taken absolutely regularly, started 1 week before entering infected areas, continued while there and for 4–6 weeks after leaving.

Laboratory diagnosis of malaria

The four species of *Plasmodium* which may give rise to malaria in man have essentially the same life-cycle, and since they are transmitted by the same vectors it might seem only of academic interest to be able to distinguish one species from another. However, the different species, and different strains of the same species, differ markedly in their epidemiological behaviour. More importantly, since the different species affect the human host differently, and since they respond differently to treatment, it is essential to be able to distinguish them at all stages of development.

Various serological techniques have been developed for the study of malaria parasites, but these are probably of little value in routine hospital work. The only certain method of diagnosing malaria — or rather of identifying the species of malaria in a human infection — is by finding the parasites. The usual (and probably the simplest and most effective) method is to examine thick or thin blood films stained with one of the Romanowsky stains. The parasites in such a film are dead, and have been distorted considerably during the drying of the blood film, and only slightly resemble the living parasites. Nevertheless, the forms shown by the different species are characteristic, and fairly easy to distinguish.

Identification of species of malaria in thin blood films

Malaria parasites are more easily identified in thin blood films than in thick blood films, because in thin films the erythrocytes are visible and frame the parasites. The malaria parasites, when correctly stained with a Romanowsky stain, have deep red nuclei and blue cytoplasm.

Plasmodium falciparum (see Fig. 2.2)
The very young trophozoite, or 'ring' form, appears as a small fine ring of cyto-plasm, less than 2 μm in diameter, with the chromatin protruding from the ring in one or two dots or as a longer bar. The central 'vacuole' may be white, or may show the pink colour of the erythrocyte. Sometimes the parasite is arranged on the periphery of the erythrocyte, when it is known as an 'accole' or 'applique' form. Multiple infections of erythrocytes are common. The infection at this stage may be overlooked because the parasites are so fine and may be in small numbers.

Within about 18 hours the ring has enlarged to about 4 μm in diameter, with thicker cytoplasm. The parasitized erythrocytes are normal in size or perhaps smaller, but they may show coarse, irregular purplish markings known as 'Maurer's spots'. There may be some small protrustions of cytoplasm from the periphery of the ring, and occasionally the rings may take on bizarre forms, but there is no marked amoeboid development as in *P. vivax*. The so-called 'tenue forms' are long filamentous parasites which may be found in India and certain parts of Africa, and are atypical amoeboid parasites.

A few hours later the vacuole begins to disappear, and small pigment granules may be seen. At this stage the ring forms disappear from the peripheral blood.

The remainder of the asexual cycle normally occurs only in the blood vessels of the internal organs, although prolonged search may reveal occasional schizonts in the peripheral blood. The prevalence of such schizonts varies in different geographical localities, but generally they are most commonly found in intense infections or terminal infections. The mature schizont normally contains 8–24 merozoites, and is in a normal-sized erythrocyte.

About 10–14 days after the ring forms first appear in the blood, large numbers of fully grown gametocytes appear in the circulation. These gametocytes differ from all other stages of human malaria parasites in that they are typically sausage-shaped — although they are generally referred to as 'crescents'. The fully developed gametocyte is longer than an erythrocyte, and the enclosing cell is stretched across the concavity of the parasite and not normally visible. The gametocyte has a central nucleus and contains a large amount of pigment. The male or microgametocyte has pale pinkish-blue cytoplasm with the blackish-brown pigment distributed through it, and a central diffuse large pink nucleus. The female or macrogametocyte has dark blue cytoplasm with the pigment collected together round the compact central nucleus. These 'crescents' are diagnostic of *P. falciparum*.

Very fine ring forms suggest *P. falciparum*, but differences in appearance between ring forms of different species of malaria are slight; and it is not possible to identify the species of malaria if only a small number of ring forms are seen. However, the presence of large numbers of ring forms, either alone or with 'crescents' only, is diagnostic of *P. falciparum*.

Plasmodium vivax (see Fig. 2.2)

The first stage to appear in the peripheral blood is the ring form. In the very early stages the rings are rather like those of *P. falciparum*, although multiple infections and accole forms are uncommon. Within a few hours the rings become larger and 'heavier-looking', tending to be thickened at one side with the nucleus at the other, and may show amoeboid processes and some yellow or brown pigment granules. The parasite later becomes irregular in shape because it is very active in an amoeboid manner (hence the name *vivax*). These changes in the parasite are accompanied by changes in the erythrocyte, which becomes larger and paler and usually shows stippling with fine regular pink spots known as 'Schuffner's dots'. This enlargement and stippling of the parasitized erythrocyte is present throughout the remainder of the asexual cycle, and is an important recognition point. After about 36 hours the parasite has grown to the size of the original erythrocyte, but it does not fill the cell because the erythrocyte has also enlarged. At this stage the parasite may be of almost any shape, and the vacuole which is present in the ring form has disappeared.

The parasite then rounds off, the nucleus divides, and part of the cytoplasm collects round each nucleus so that the parasite comes to consist of about 16 merozoites (the number may vary from 12–24). These merozoites, about 2 μm in size, split off and become arranged around the central mass which consists of left-over cytoplasm and malarial pigment. The distended erythrocyte then disrupts, and the merozoites are released into the circulation, where they enter fresh blood cells.

Gametocytes usually appear in the peripheral blood within the first week after blood forms first appear. The gametocytes are about the same size as schizonts, but differ from schizonts in having a single nucleus and pigment that is scattered throughout the cytoplasm of the parasite. The differences between the sexes are of no practical importance, but the macrogametocyte (female) has darker and more deeply stained cytoplasm, and the nucleus tends to be smaller and more compact, than that of the microgametocyte (male).

Plasmodium malariae (see Fig. 2.2)

The small trophozoites (ring forms) which first appear in the blood are stout rings that measure about one-third of the diameter of the erythrocyte, with the chromatin dot or nucleus on the circumference of the ring. The vacuole of the ring form is often discoloured, so that the ring shape is not very obvious. When it grows the parasite tends to assume an elongated form, and the large trophozoites are not the flimsy amoeboid structures seen in *P. vivax* but have a much more solid and compact appearance. The cytoplasm tends to stain dark blue, and often assumes the shape of a broad belt across the circumference of the erythrocyte, with the chromatin drawn out into a line on one side and the pigment on the opposite side. This is known as the 'band form'. The pigment is dark yellow or brown, and occurs in coarse granules. The pigment is formed early, usually after about 12 hours.

After 48 hours the parasite occupies the greater part of the erythrocyte, which is not enlarged. Nuclear division may have commenced after 48 hours, and by 60 hours segmentation is relatively well advanced. The full asexual cycle takes 72 hours, and after this period the mature schizonts are formed. The schizont contains 8–12 merozoites arranged in a rosette around a central mass of cytoplasm and pigment. The merozoites are smaller and more intensely staining than those of *P. vivax*, and the pigment is markedly coarse.

The gametocytes are smaller and more deeply stained than those of *P. vivax*. The parasitized erythrocytes are unchanged in size, although they may be a little darker in colour. Stippling does not occur, though occasionally a few dark-coloured spots known as 'Ziemann's dots' may be seen, especially if the staining is heavy. The microgametocyte takes stain more lightly than the macrogametocyte, and is smaller than the macrogametocyte, with the chromatin diffused and sometimes stretched out in the form of a belt. The mature macrogametocyte completely fills the erythrocyte, and stains deeply, with the chromatin compact and eccentric.

Plasmodium ovale (see Fig. 2.2)

The asexual forms resemble those of *P. malariae* in that the cytoplasm is deeply staining, often occurring in band forms, and that the pigment is coarse and dark. They differ from those of *P. malariae* in that the infected erythrocyte usually exhibits Schuffner's dots, and may be slightly enlarged. The young ring forms of *P. ovale* are more dense and solid-looking than those of either *P. vivax* or *P. falciparum*, and amoeboid activity is very limited. There is a relatively large amount of chromatin which is often irregularly shaped. As the parasite develops, brown pigment appears and the red cell enlarges to some extent. There is a very early development of stippling, and a large proportion of the infected red cells may show ragged edges. When the parasite is half grown the chromatin begins to divide, and at this stage the parasite is most easy to recognize because about 25 per cent of the infected red cells have an oval shape, often with fimbriated (fringed) edges at one or both poles. The parasite is not oval but rounded, and is about the size of the normal red cell. When schizogony is completed there are about eight merozoites arranged around a central pigment mass. The sexual forms are indistinguishable from those of *P. malariae* except for the decolourized red blood cell, the presence of Schuffner's dots, and possibly the shape of the red blood cell.

Stippling of infected erythrocytes
The importance of stippling of the infected erythrocytes is frequently misunderstood. The presence of Shuffner's dots is sure evidence that the causal organism is either *P.vivax* or *P. ovale*, while the presence of Maurer's spots is similarly proof of *P. falciparum* infection. The absence of stippling proves nothing. The stippling is, so to speak, a trick of the stain, and it may be absent from a poorly stained blood film and present in a better-stained film made from the same patient at the same time.

Identification of species of malaria in thick blood films

Malaria parasites are more difficult to recognize in thick blood films because the erythrocytes have been lysed and therefore the parasites are not clearly 'framed' by them. Nevertheless, thick blood films are increasingly used in diagnosis because such films permit the rapid examination of much larger volumes of blood than do thin blood films, and so enable more rapid diagnosis, especially when there is only a light parasitaemia.

Only a small part of a thick blood film will be correctly stained, because differences in the thickness of different parts of the film produce differences in degree of dehaemoglobinization, in staining, and in other factors. When examining thick blood films stained with Romanowsky stains, it is essential to select a part of the film that is polychromatically stained. This part can be recognized because in it the nuclei of the leucocytes are stained a rich purple colour.

For identification of the different species of malaria it is necessary to recognize both the stages present and the appearance of these stages. The characteristics that enable identification of the species are as follows.

Plasmodium falciparum
The stages present will be 'ring' forms only (they may be small, large or of both kinds), 'ring' forms and 'crescents' (gametocytes), or if the patient has taken a schizonticidal drug, 'crescents' only. The 'ring' forms may be turned or twisted

at various angles, and so appear in various unusual shapes such as 'comma forms', 'exclamation mark forms', and 'propeller forms'.

Plasmodium vivax
'Ring' forms may be present, but these are not specifically identifiable. The older trophozoites are markedly amoeboid, and so very irregular in shape. The schizonts and gametocytes are about as large as lymphocytes. Occasionally lysed infected erythrocytes may be stained a pale pink colour and appear as 'ghost cells', or Shuffner's dots may outline the position of lysed erythrocytes.

Plasmodium malariae
'Ring' forms may be present, but these are not specifically identifiable. The older trophozoites are small and solid, and deeply stained. The fully grown parasites are smaller than lymphocytes (but occasionally a ruptured schizont may appear to be as large as a lymphocyte). The pigment granules in the parasites are dark, coarse and profuse.

Plasmodium ovale
This species can rarely be identified with certainty in thick blood films. The 'solidity' of the parasites and the presence of coarse pigment granules suggest *P. malariae*. Pink staining of some of the lysed infected erythrocytes and the presence of Shuffner's dots suggest *P. vivax* (but Shuffner's dots do not always stain in thick blood films). A tentative diagnosis of *P. ovale* must be confirmed by examination of a thin blood film.

Before leaving the subject of the laboratory diagnosis of malaria, a word of warning must be given concerning mixed infections. Such infections are by no means uncommon, and it cannot be too strongly emphasized that the demonstration of one, or even two, species of malaria in the blood is no guarantee that another, and possibly more dangerous, species may not also be present. And although the finding of the parasites is the only certain laboratory method of diagnosing malaria, the failure to find parasites in a blood smear cannot justify a confident statement that malaria is absent if clinical signs are present. Nevertheless, although the examination of a negative thick blood film may not rule out malaria, it is certainly suggestive.

Control of malaria

Eradication of malaria has been possible in Europe and North America, but has proved very difficult in most areas of Africa, Asia and South America where vector anopheline mosquitoes can survive more easily. A combination of methods aimed at controlling vectors and protecting recipients is necessary.

Drainage or chemical treatment of anopheline breeding sites is basic. The antimalarial campaigns in the 1950s and the 1960s were largely based on house spraying with residual insecticides. However, developing anopheline resistance to insecticides, the change of resting and biting habits to outside houses (exophily), and economic difficulties, contributed to the ultimate failure of many of these campaigns.

Other features of control include mass chemotherapy, detection and treatment of cases, and prolonged supervision of the situation after attempts at anopheline control. On a more individual basis chemoprophylaxis, and protection against mosquito bites by the use of bed nets, screening of houses, and wearing long-sleeved clothes and long trousers when out after dark, are important.

Resistance of malaria parasites to chloroquine has greatly complicated the situation. The WHO has abandoned the concept of universal malaria eradication as impracticable at the moment, but aims at reduction of the morbidity and mortality caused by malaria by widespread provision of treatment facilities in the community. Research continues in attempts to produce antimalarial vaccines.

The Coccidia

These are a group of parasites that are common in animals and are sometimes of considerable veterinary importance, but they are not frequently found in man. They have life-cycles which, on the whole, are similar to those of the malaria parasites, except that typically they pass the whole of their life in the cells of the intestinal wall of their host, apart from a free-living period during which the infective stages are carried to a new host.

Some of the coccidia can be found in the deeper organs of their hosts, and a few have complicated life-cycles that involve intermediate hosts. Among the latter are *Sarcocystis* and *Toxoplasma*, and man may harbour the asexual stages of both these parasites. *Sarcocystis* infections in man are usually chance findings, and seem to be of no clinical significance, but *Toxoplasma* causes infections that may be fatal. Other pathogenic coccidia, about which relatively little is known, are *Pneumocystis* and *Cryptosporidium*.

Isospora belli

Isospora belli, which is widespread throughout the world but only occasionally reported in man, is a typical coccidian. Development occurs in the epithelial cells of the villi of the small intestine, but the only stage normally seen is the oocyst which occurs in the faeces. This oocyst is a transparent, usually ovoid, body, about 30 μm by 12 μm, and containing a spherical zygote. Maturation takes place outside the host's body, and the mature infective oocyst contains eight sporozoites.

Infection in man is usually associated with diarrhoea, usually lasting for two to three weeks but sometimes persisting for months or years. Many infections are asymptomatic, and rarely serious illness may result, possibly associated with immunological deficiency of the infected individual.

Toxoplasma gondii

Toxoplasma has been recorded in a wide variety of hosts, including man, various domestic and wild mammals, and birds; and in all these animals the same species, *T. gondii*, is involved. The trophozoite stage occurs in the cells of the reticuloendothelial system, and the encysted stage occurs in the cells of various organs, mainly the muscles and brain. The unencysted parasites are rather crescent-shaped, about 5 μm long and 2.5 μm wide, with one end more pointed than the other. In the early acute stages of infection these parasites (or 'tachyzoites') are usually found in the phagocytic cells of various internal organs, and in mononuclear leucocytes. In chronic infections the parasites appear as more rounded bodies (or 'bradyzoites') which multiply within the cells of host organs, usually in muscle or brain, to produce cysts. These are all asexual stages of the parasite.

The infection in man is essentially at a dead end, although tachyzoites can pass across the placenta to the fetus during pregnancy. If an animal harbouring the asexual stages is eaten by a carnivore other than a cat, the encysted stages develop into tachyzoites and produce an acute infection, which then proceeds to a chronic infection with encysted parasites. If an animal harbouring the encysted stages is eaten by a cat, a typical coccidian development takes place in the wall of the cat's intestine. The final stage of this development is an 'oocyst' that is passed in the faeces and develops to maturity on the ground. If the developed oocyst is eaten by a herbivorous animal (including man) an asexual infection will develop.

Human infection can thus result from ingestion of oocysts from cat faeces, from ingestion of encysted stages in the meat of domestic animals, or by transplacental transmission.

Medical aspects of toxoplasmosis

Pathogenesis

Toxoplasms released from cysts in enterocytes are carried in the blood and lymphatic systems (probably within leucocytes) to many organs. The brain, retina, myocardium, muscles, lungs and liver are all likely to be invaded. Cellular invasion and intracellular toxoplasmal multiplication cause cell destruction, liberation of parasites that invade neighbouring cells, and necrotic foci leading to marked local cellular inflammatory reactions. In an immunocompetent individual this destructive process is rapidly halted by immune processes, and the disease is minimal or subclinical. In the fetus and in immunocompromised hosts the pathological process is not arrested, and necrotizing encephalitis, pneumonitis and hepatitis result. In the brain there is necrosis, glial cell proliferation and perivascular lymphocytic infiltration which may result in aqueductal obstruction and hydrocephalus in congenital infections.

An unusual feature of toxoplasmosis is that the organisms persist in cysts in various organs for the remainder of the infected person's life. Dormant cysts are the probable source of organisms that cause serious invasive disease after damage to the immune system in later life, and relapsing choroidoretinitis in children and adults.

Immunity

Because of the intracellular habitat of the organisms, cell-mediated immunity is of great importance. Immune sensitization of lymphocytes induces production of lymphokines which prevents intracellular multiplication of the parasites in macrophages and other cells. Humoral antibodies may have some effect on parasites during brief periods of extracellular existence. IgM antibodies are an indication of recent infection and do not persist; IgG antibodies reach their peak about two months after infection and persist for many years. Specific IgG and IgM can be measured by indirect immunofluorescence. Normally, immunity to toxoplasmosis is life-long.

Clinical features

There are no specific manifestations of toxoplasmosis, and the clinical features of the infection vary widely according to the immune status of the patient.

Acquired toxoplasmosis in the immunocompetent host
Usually the disease is subclinical, and only diagnosable from the appearance of antibodies. The most common clinical manifestation is enlargement of lymphatic glands, particularly the cervical ones. In about half of these patients there are other symptoms such as fever, malaise and sore throat, and less commonly a maculopapular skin rash. The lymphadenopathy may persist for weeks or months, but symptoms gradually resolve spontaneously. Rarely serious complications such as pneumonitis, myocarditis, meningoencephalitis and hepatitis occur, alone or in combination, and these can prove fatal if not treated.

Congenital infection
The fetus is at risk if a woman acquires a primary toxoplasmal infection during pregnancy. This may occur in about 0.5 per cent of pregnancies in Europe, and about 40 per cent of the fetuses are affected. Neurological involvement of the fetus can result in necrotizing encephalitis with hydrocephalus, microcephaly, mental retardation, epilepsy, intracranial calcification and choroidoretinitis. There may also be pneumonitis, hepatitis, hepatosplenomegaly, jaundice and a maculopapular rash. The infection may be fatal.

Ocular involvement
Ocular involvement usually arises, as a late manifestation of congenital infection, in childhood or adult life, and the damage is probably immunologically mediated. Less commonly, choroidoretinitis occurs during the acute stage of congenital or acquired infection. Toxoplasmosis has been estimated to be the cause of 30 per cent of choroidoretinitis in children.

Active lesions can cause blurred vision, ocular pain and epiphora. Strabismus may be an early symptom in children. Macular involvement causes loss of central vision. Recurrent flare-ups result in progressive destruction of retinal tissue and sometimes glaucoma. On fundoscopy, acute lesions are yellowish-white and elevated; older lesions show white plaques with black areas of choroidal pigmentation.

Toxoplasmosis in the immunocompromised host
This is an 'opportunist' infection. If cell-mediated immunity is impaired in AIDS, lymphoma, or in patients on immunosuppressive drugs, there may be a breakdown of old toxoplasma lesions, or possibly a new infection. The resulting

illness progresses rapidly and can end fatally. Central nervous involvement is the commonest presentation, with symptoms of meningoencephalitis or focal pathology. Headache, mental deterioration, and seizures or symptoms of a cerebral mass lesion, may all occur, with changes in the cerebrospinal fluid.

Diagnosis

Diagnosis depends on serological tests. In suspected cases tests for IgG (dye tests or complement fixation tests) and for IgM (indirect immunofluorescence) should be performed. High titres of 1:1000 or more, and the presence of IgM antibodies, suggest recent infections, and rising titres 2 weeks later are conclusive.

Toxoplasmal IgM antibodies in cord blood are conclusive evidence of congenital infection, but they are only present in 25 per cent of such cases. In suspected cases of congenital infection, IgG levels of toxoplasmal antibodies should be followed up after birth.

Treatment

Toxoplasmosis does not require treatment in immunocompetent people with lymphadenitis alone. Toxoplasmosis should be treated in subjects with impaired immunity, in those with choroidoretinitis, and during pregnancy.

In adults, pyrimethamine 75 mg is given as a loading dose, and then 25 mg daily is given for one month. In addition sulphadiazine is given in 6-hourly doses of 1 g for the same time, together with folinic acid 5–10 mg daily to prevent marrow damage by the pyrimethamine. Infants' doses of pyrimethamine are 1 mg/kg per day for 3 days and then 0.5 mg/kg per day for 4 weeks; the dose of sulphadiazine is 100 mg/kg per day in 4 doses for 4 weeks. These drugs are hazardous for the fetus in the first 3 months of pregnancy, and spiramycin 2 g daily in 4 doses for 3 weeks is preferred in pregnancy. This course should be repeated until term, with 2 weeks' rest periods between courses.

Prevention

Quite a high proportion of mutton and pork products contain infective cysts of *Toxoplasma*. Proper cooking of meat, to a temperature of at least 60°C, will destroy the cysts. It is also important that hands are washed after handling uncooked meat.

At least 1 per cent of cats excrete infective oocysts in their faeces. There is danger of contaminating one's hands when cleaning out cats' sleeping boxes or other places where cats rest, and gloves should be worn during such cleaning.

Avoidance of infection is particularly important in pregnancy.

Pneumocystis carinii

Pneumocystis is now generally accepted as a protozoan related to the coccidia, although it has been grouped with the amoebae and with the fungi. The trophozoite stage appears to be a protozoan but the cysts resemble some fungi. Both stages occur in the pulmonary alveoli of their hosts, which include man, rodents, guinea pigs and other mammals in most countries of the world. The cyst is about 5 μm in diameter and contains up to eight bodies known as 'sporozoites'. The 'trophozoite', which is possibly an excysted 'sporozoite', is rather amoeboid and up to 4 μm in diameter.

The basic life-cycle of *P. carinii* is only incompletely known; the mode of transmission is doubtful, but both contagious and airborne transmission have been suggested. Infection causes pneumonitis (and sometimes death) in severely undernourished individuals, especially children.

Medical aspects of pneumocystosis

Pathogenesis

Pneumocystis carinii has been found in the lungs of man and animals without respiratory troubles, and 75 per cent of children aged 4 years show serological evidence of previous infection. Serious pneumonitis seems to occur only in immunosuppressed hosts. Many causes of immunosuppression have been associated with *P. carinii* pneumonia, including neoplasia (especially lymphomas), immunosuppressive drugs, congenital immune deficient syndromes, acquired immune deficiency syndrome, protein calorie deficiency and aplastic anaemia. *Pneumocystis* pneumonia is often also accompanied by other bacterial or viral infections.

Pathological changes include heavy infiltration and thickening of the alveolar septa with plasma cells and lymphocytes, desquamation of alveolar lining cells, and extensive foamy exudate in the alveoli. This exudate consists of desquamated cells, parasites, mononuclear cells and proteinaceous fluid. The changes are bilateral, spreading extensively from the hila to mid and lower zones; pleural involvement is uncommon, and spread outside the lungs is very rare. The functional result is interference with oxygen diffusion and hypoxia with normal carbon dioxide tensions. Recovery from the acute illness is usually associated with resolution of pulmonary changes, but pulmonary fibrosis occasionally results.

Clinical picture

The respiratory illness may be preceded by coryza or diarrhoea, as well as other signs produced by the cause of the immune deficiency. Tachypnoea and dry unproductive cough are the commonest symptoms. In late cases physical examination reveals diffuse crepitations on auscultation; and chest X-ray will show extensive bilateral alveolar exudation, most marked in middle and lower zones. Fever is present in children but not prominent in adults. The arterial oxygen falls with an arterial pO_2 of less than 80 mm Hg; cyanosis appears later as the disease evolves over the course of 1–3 weeks. Untreated, the illness is usually fatal; but with cotrimoxazole the mortality rate has been reduced to about 25 per cent, although some patients will have subsequent attacks.

The organism is of low virulence, but the infection can spread in nurseries and orphanages among poorly nourished children. Spread to the fetus has also been reported.

Diagnosis

There are many possible differential diagnoses including bacterial, mycotic and cytomegalovirus infections.

Definitive diagnosis depends on microscopic identification of the organism, preferably after obtaining bronchial exudate by endobronchial brush biopsy. Bronchial aspiration and tracheal lavage have been less successful. Open or needle lung biopsy is often diagnostic, but is more hazardous.

Serological methods using indirect immunofluorescence or the complement fixation test are not very reliable.

Treatment and prevention

Specific treatment
Trimethoprim/sulphamethoxazole (co-trimoxazole) is given in doses of trimethoprim 20 mg/kg per day and sulphamethoxazole 100 mg/kg per day in 4 daily doses for 14 days. If the patient does not respond, the second-choice drug is pentamidine isethionate in doses of 4 mg/kg per day, given as a singular intramuscular injection daily for 14 days. Co-trimoxazole is preferred to pentamidine because the latter is more toxic, giving rise to nephrotoxic, hepatotoxic, haematological effects and causing hypoglycaemia.

Supportive treatment
Many patients will need oxygen therapy at a concentration of not more than 50 volumes per cent to keep the pO_2 above 70 mm Hg. If this oxygen pressure cannot be maintained, assisted ventilation is indicated. Immunosuppressive drugs should be discontinued if possible.

Prevention
Trimethoprim 5 mg/kg per day and suphamethoxazole 25 mg/kg per day in 2 divided doses daily prevent pneumocystis pneumonia in susceptible patients.

Cryptosporidium

Cryptosporidium was first described in a mouse, and various species have now been reported from reptiles, birds and mammals — the one in man has been named *C. garnhami*. Infections in man are often in immunologically deficient or immunologically compromised individuals. It seems probable that human infection is zoonotic, man being infected by oocysts from cattle faeces, but some authorities consider the various species of *Cryptosporidium* to be host specific.

Development occurs in the brush border of the gastric or intestinal mucosal epithelium, and all stages of the parasite are 6 μm or less in diameter. Oocysts containing four sporozoites have been found in faeces, but the method of transmission has not yet been clarified.

Cryptosporidiosis

Cryptosporidiosis has long been known to cause diarrhoea in calves and other animals, and now that it is being systematically sought in human faeces, it has been identified as a not uncommon human infection. In immunocompetent hosts, parasites are usually found in the stools of young children with watery diarrhoea of mild or moderate severity. Some excretors of the organisms are asymptomatic. In subjects with the acquired immune deficiency syndrome, however, infection can cause a prolonged, severe watery diarrhoea with abdominal cramps, wasting and fever. No effective treatment is known, but the use of spiramycin is under trial.

Further reading

Bruce-Chwatt LJ. *Essential malariology*. London: Heinemann, 1980.
Cohen S (ed). Malaria. *Br Med Bull* 1982; **38**: 115–218.
Garnham PCC. *Malaria Parasites and Other Haemosporidia*. Oxford: Blackwell, 1966.
Harrison G. *Mosquitoes, malaria and Man*. London: John Murray, 1978.
McGregor IA. Current concepts concerning man's resistance to malaria. *Bull Soc Pathologie Exotique* 1983; **76**: 433–45.
Spencer HC, Strickland GT. Malaria. In: Strickland GT (ed) *Hunter's tropical medicine*, 6th edn., Philadelphia: Saunders, 1984.
White NJ, Warrell DA. Clinical management of chloroquine-resistant *Plasmodium falciparum* malaria in southeast Asia. *Tropical Doctor* 1983; **13**: 153–58.

3

Trypanosomes

The flagellates that parasitize the blood and various tissues in man are called haemoflagellates. The blood-inhabiting forms live in the plasma, not the red blood cells. These parasites are of the family Trypanosomatidae, and belong to the two genera *Trypanosoma* and *Leishmania*. They may cause serious and often fatal disease in man. The genus *Trypanosoma* is responsible for trypanosomiasis, the African form which is commonly but rather misleadingly called 'sleeping sickness' and the American form is called Chagas' disease. The genus *Leishmania* is responsible for the visceral and cutaneous forms of leishmaniasis known respectively as kala-azar and tropical sore. The genus *Leishmania* differs from the genus *Trypanosoma* in that its members do not exhibit a undulating membrane at any stage in their development (see chapter 4).

Trypanosoma

Members of this genus have been found parasitizing all types of vertebrates, both warm- and cold-blooded, and have a world-wide distribution. Trypanosomes occurring in animals in temperate countries (with one notable exception in *T. equiperdum*) are usually responsible only for inapparent infections and appear to cause little disturbance to their host. In distinction to this, many of the trypanosomes occurring in the tropics are highly pathogenic. There are two sub-species, *T. brucei gambiense* and *T. b. rhodesiense*, which cause widespread endemic disease (sleeping sickness) in Africa south of the Sahara, and one species, *T cruzi*, which causes widespread disease (Chagas' disease) in Central and South America.

A trypanosome is elongated, flattened and somewhat lancet-shaped. It has a single nucleus of the vesicular type containing a large central karyosome (which is only seen after 'wet fixation' of specimens). In dried films stained by the Romanowsky method the nucleus appears to be filled with irregular granules. There is a single flagellum that arises at the posterior end of the body and runs to the anterior end, along the outer margin of an outgrowth of the pellicle that extends along the whole length of the body. This outgrowth is known as the undulating membrane, and serves to propel the trypanosome in the same way as a fin propels a fish. The flagellum may extend beyond the anterior end of the body and the undulating membrane as a 'free' flagellum. The flagellum arises from a basal body situated near a conspicuous round or rod-shaped organelle known as the kinetoplast.

Multiplication of trypanosomes is by longitudinal fission, the process beginning by division of the kinetoplast. Next the nucleus divides, and then the trypanosome divides longitudinally to form two separate protozoans. There is apparently no sexual reproduction.

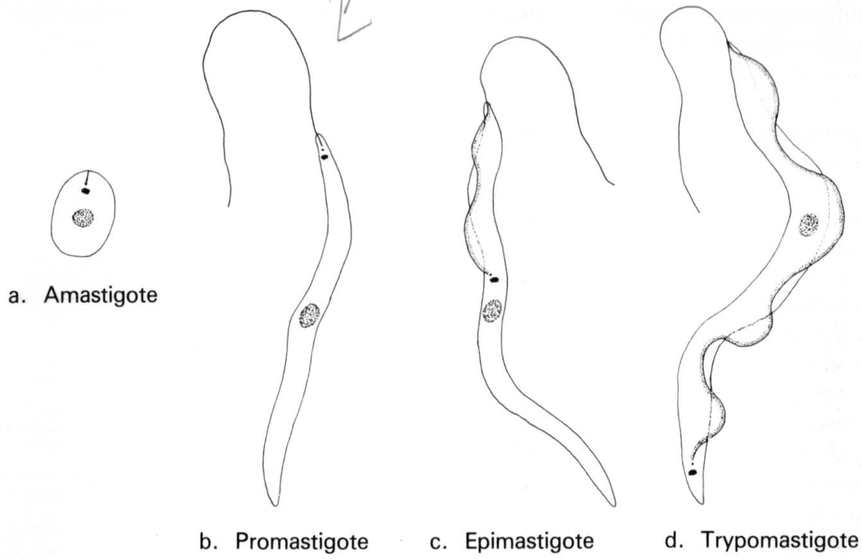

a. Amastigote

b. Promastigote   c. Epimastigote   d. Trypomastigote

Fig. 3.1 Developmental forms of Haemoflagellates.

During the life-cycle there are four stages through which the parasites may pass. These are:

1. The amastigote (Fig. 3.1a). The body is spherical or ovoid and about half the size of a red blood cell. The kinetoplast is near the nucleus. There is no flagellum or undulating membrane.
2. The promastigote (Fig. 3.1b). The body is elongated. The kinetoplast and the origin of the flagellum are well in front of the nucleus. A free flagellum is present.
3. The epimastigote (Fig. 3.1c). The body is elongated. The kinetoplast and the origin of the flagellum are close to (usually just in front of) the nucleus. Hence there is only a short length of undulating membrane. A free flagellum is usually present.
4. The trypomastigote.(Fig. 3.1d). The body is elongated. The kinetoplast and the origin of the flagellum are well behind the nucleus, near the posterior end of the body. There may or may not be a free flagellum.

African trypanosomiasis

T. b. gambiense and *T. b. rhodesiense* are transmitted by the same insect vector, the tsetse fly (*Glossina*) and are morphologically indistinguishable in the human host and in their developmental stages in the insect vector. They are also indistinguishable from *T. b. brucei* in animals. These three trypanosomes can be regarded as three biological races belonging to one and the same species. However, since they occur in different hosts, differ in the types of disease produced, and differ in their general biological features, it is convenient to refer to them under separate specific names. The nature of the trypanosomes in natural infections is determined largely on circumstantial grounds provided by epidemiological data. *T. b. brucei* cannot infect man, and *T. b. rhodesiense* resembles it more than does *T. b. gambiense*, so it seems probable that evolution has been from *T. b. brucei* to *T. b. rhodesiense* to *T. b gambiense*.

African trypanosomiasis or sleeping sickness occurs in tropical Africa between 15°N and 15°S. *T. b. gambiense* occurs mainly in West and Central Africa, southern Sudan and Uganda. *T. b. rhodesiense* occurs in East and East Central Africa, from Ethiopia to Botswana. The different distributions depend on the distributions of the respective vector species of tsetse flies and in some parts of Africa the distributions of the two sub-species overlap.

It is convenient to begin consideration of the life-cycle at the stage when the infective trypanosome is injected by the biting insect. This infective stage is injected with the saliva of the fly before the fly commences to feed. Parasites that have reached their infective stage of development in the salivary glands or mouthparts of the vector, and that are inoculated into the host during the act of biting, are referred to as being in the 'anterior station', in distinction from parasites that reach their final stage of development in the gut of the vector and are transmitted to the host in the faeces, which are referred to as being in the 'posterior station'. The infective forms of the malaria parasite in the mosquito and of the trypanosome in the tsetse are both in the 'anterior station'.

Trypanosomiasis is transmissible by direct inoculation with a needle, provided that the transfer is made before the death of the parasite. This type of transmission may theoretically occur with any biting insect whose mouthparts are sufficiently coarse to carry an infective dose of blood during interrupted feeding, and it is referred to as 'mechanical', as distinct from 'cyclical' transmission in which the parasite completes a cycle of development before being capable of infecting a new host. The tsetse fly has comparatively coarse mouthparts, and is a mechanical as well as a cyclical vector of both human and animal trypanosomiasis. Most transmission is cyclical.

The trypanosomes that are inoculated into the subcutaneous tissues by the biting tsetse develop and multiply at the site of injection, and their presence often causes a local inflammation, sometimes referred to as a 'chancre', which resolves spontaneously. The chancre only follows the bite of an infective fly. A further 1–3 weeks elapse before the trypanosomes have invaded the peripheral blood in sufficient numbers to be detected by direct examination. Periodic disappearance occurs, and trypanosomes may be absent from the blood for some months in old-standing cases. About the time the trypanosomes appear in the blood, in most cases, the lymphatic glands become involved, but only in very late infections are trypanosomes found in the cerebrospinal fluid. The symptoms produced when they are in the cerebrospinal fluid give rise to the popular name of 'sleeping sickness'. In all these anatomical sites the trypanosomes have the same morphological appearance. The size of the trypanosomes is of little value as a guide to the recognition of species, since it varies not only with the species but also in individual members of the same species.

African trypanosomes are pleomorphic, and the trypanosomes found in the blood differ considerably in size and shape, in the presence or absence of a free flagellum, and in other details. There is usually a mixture of long slender forms, short stumpy forms and intermediate forms.

T. b. rhodesiense is transmitted by the '*morsitans* group' of tsetse flies, which live in the savannah woodlands of East and Central Africa. The flies also feed on wild animals, especially antelopes, and *T. b. rhodesiense* causes a zoonotic infection that usually produces acute disease in man. *T. b. gambiense* is transmitted by the '*palpalis* group' of tsetse flies, which live mainly in the vegetation alongside rivers, lakes and other permanent water in West Africa. The disease produced by *T. b. gambiense* is chronic, the parasite has been found in various domestic animals, but there is no proof that any of these are reservoir hosts for the human infection.

The feeding fly sucks up blood, and any contained trypanosomes pass into the mid-gut where they are enclosed in the 'peritrophic membrane'. Many of the trypanosomes in the lumen of the insect's gut are digested, but the remainder develop; it has been suggested that only the stumpy forms will develop in the fly. The trypanosomes multiply intensely, and about the fourth day after ingestion they enter the space between the peritrophic membrane and the wall of the mid-gut, and they develop there to produce large numbers of thin trypomastigote forms. The remainder of the cycle in the fly is not known definitely, but the slender mid-gut forms finally enter the salivary glands, where they complete their development. They are transformed into 'metacyclic trypanosomes' which are small, with or without a flagellum, like the stumpy blood forms. Only the metacyclic forms are infective to the mammalian host. The cycle in the tsetse fly takes 15–35 days, and the fly remains infective for the remainder of its life, which may be several months.

Gambiense trypanosomiasis

Pathogenesis

In some patients the initial manifestation is a local subcutaneous swelling or chancre appearing a few days after an infective tsetse bite at the site of the bite. The chancre is an inflammatory reaction to locally multiplying trypanosomes. Resolution occurs within two weeks, but the parasites reach the blood stream either directly or via the lymphatics. There follows a chronic intermittent parasitaemia lasting months or even years, which is associated with general symptoms such as fever, wasting and anaemia. Eventually, within 6–18 months or occasionally after some years, the central nervous system is invaded, producing a chronic meningoencephalitis that is fatal unless treated.

Tissue damage is probably largely immunologically mediated. Immune complexes are formed, kinins and pyrogens are liberated and inflammatory changes occur in various tissues. Parasites of *T. b. gambiense* can change their surface antigens up to 20 times by a genetic switch mechanism. The consequences of this are evasion of immune destruction by the host, massive proliferation of B lymphocytes and considerable production of immunoglobulin M with high serum levels of IgM. There is moderate autoimmune haemolysis and also thrombocytopenia. There is a generalized hyperplasia of the reticuloendothelial system including lymph glands and spleen.

Penetration of the blood–brain barrier by the trypanosomes results in a chronic meningoencephalitis with perivascular cuffing of cerebral vessels by lymphocytes, neuronal destruction, gliosis and demyelination. Neurological involvement is associated with CSF changes — increased protein (including

IgM) content, a lymphocytic pleocytosis and sometimes the presence of trypanosomes.

Immunity

There is a vigorous humoral response to infection with trypanosomes, large amounts of IgM and some autoantibodies are produced, but the immune response fails to eliminate the infection, possibly because of antigenic variation. However, when the disease has been present in a particular area for a long time the local people appear more resistant to the disease than people in a newly affected area. Trypanosomiasis causes a degree of immune suppression to bacterial infections that often complicates the late stage of the disease and may cause death.

Clinical aspects

Early stages

European patients often note the presence of a local, mildly painful, subcutaneous swelling, commonly on the arm or face, appearing a few days after a tsetse bite. Many indigenous victims either do not have or do not notice the initial chancre. The swelling resolves spontaneously within two weeks, and may be associated with local lymph gland swelling. Fever may appear whilst the chancre is still present. The usual incubation period before generalized symptoms is about 2 weeks, but is sometimes delayed for months or rarely years. Irregular fever continues for months or years; it may occur in bouts lasting days or weeks, then disappear for weeks at a time. Headache is prominent; and wasting, anaemia, and splenomegaly are found. During the first few months transient, scattered areas of subcutaneous oedema occur. In Europeans circinate, erythematous rashes are seen, particularly on the back and trunk. These signs are regarded as due to local hypersensitivity reactions to products of the trypanosomes. Generalized enlargement of superficial lymph nodes occurs, particularly noticeable in the posterior cervical region (Winterbottom's sign). The lymph nodes may enlarge periodically coinciding with febrile periods: they are rubbery initially but later fibrose and shrink.

Some cases appear mildly symptomatic for years, but eventually develop neurological trypanosomiasis. There may be a latent asymptomatic period. Usually within 6–18 months the nervous system is invaded.

Cerebral trypanosomiasis (sleeping sickness)

This chronic meningoencephalitis is invariably fatal within 12 months unless treated. Usually it follows a slowly progressive course, occasionally it is fulminant causing death in coma or in status epilepticus in a few weeks. By the time that the brain is involved the patient is afebrile. Early symptoms are increasing headache and psychological changes including apathy, depression and sometimes mania. There is progressive dementia with deteriorating social behaviour and later incontinence.

Physical symptoms include tremors, intractable itching, choreiform movements and convulsions. Gradually the patient enters the classical sleeping sickness stage in which he lapses into stupor, being unable to care for himself. Sometimes he sleeps by day and becomes restless and agitated by night. There is wasting, malnutrition and complicating infections such as pneumonia or dysentery which often prove fatal. Finally the patient drifts into irreversible coma or dies in status epilepticus.

Clinical diagnosis

The early disease must be distinguished from other causes of long continued fever with or without lymphadenopathy. These include tuberculosis, leishmaniasis and lymphoma.

Chronic meningoencephalitis in trypanosomiasis endemic areas is due to trypansomiasis in the great majority of cases, but tuberculous meningitis, subdural haematoma, cerebral tumor and neurosyphilis may need consideration as differential diagnoses.

In African trypanosomiasis, involvement of the central nervous system is assumed if the cerebrospinal protein level is increased above normal, if there are more than five leucocytes per cubic millimetre, or if both signs are present. The presure of the cerebrospinal fluid is often raised and its IgM content increased. Trypanosomes may be present in the cerebrospinal fluid, and rarely 'Mott's morular cells' are found. The latter are large, raspberry-like, plasma cells containing IgM.

Lymph node aspiration
Frequently, especially in the later stages of the disease, trypanosomes are not easily found in the blood. Examination of fluid aspirated with a dry needle and syringe from enlarged lymph glands is more likely to show trypanosomes in these cases.

Treatment

All cases of trypanosomiasis must have CSF examination to decide whether the nervous system is involved. If there is no CSF abnormality or clinical evidence of neurological involvement, suramin is given. Suramin is an acidic azo compound that binds to serum proteins and combines with parasitic enzymes. Suramin is given slowly intravenously in a test dose of 200 mg (in fresh 10 per cent solution) to test for anaphylaxis. Then five intravenous injections of 1 g are given to adults on days 1, 3, 7, 14 and 21. Suramin can cause renal damage, and the urine should be tested for protein and casts before each injection. Rarely it causes exfoliative dermititis, gastrointestinal ulceration, diarrhoea and wasting — this may be fatal. The children's dosage is 20 mg/kg for 5 injections. An alternative drug is pentamidine 4 mg/kg intramuscularly daily for 10 days.

If there is increased protein or cells in the CSF, then neurological involvement is assumed and melarsoprol (Mel B), a trivalent arsenical compound, is administered. Mel B is a highly toxic drug, sometimes causing acute reactive encephalopathy (with a high mortality rate), shock and neuropathy. It is given slowly intravenously in a 3.7 per cent solution. Various treatment regimes are used: one such is day 1, 2.5 ml; day 3, 2.5 ml; day 5, 5.0 ml; day 10, 5.0 ml; day 12,

5.0 ml; day 14, 5.0 ml; day 24, 5.0 ml; day 26, 5.0 ml; day 28, 5.0 ml; a total of 40 ml over 1 month.

BAL, the antidote for heavy-metal poisoning, may be of some use in reactive encephalopathy following MelB. Many would advocate 2–3 preliminary injections of suramin before beginning Mel B. Cases should be followed up for 1 year and lumbar puncture repeated. If relapse occurs, a further course of melarsoprol is given, and then nitrofurazone 500 mg 6-hourly for 5 days by mouth. Nitrofurazone is toxic and can cause neuropathy, mental disturbance, rashes and haemolysis in G-6-P-D deficient patients.

Rhodesiense trypanosomiasis

Pathogenesis and clinical picture

The pathogenesis of *T. b. rhodesiense* infection is basically similar to that of *T. b. gambiense*, but the parasite is less well adapted to man and causes a more virulent, rapidly progressing illness. Death often occurs within 6 months, before involvement of the nervous system. A primary chancre is more likely to be found than in *gambiense* infection, trypanosomes are more plentiful in the blood, and generalized lymphadenopathy does not usually occur. Deterioration is rapid with prostration, high fever, anaemia and wasting. Acute myocarditis is common and dangerous — cardiac failure, serious arrhythmias and sudden death may result. Small pericardial effusions are sometimes found. Hepatic damage with jaundice is seen. If the nervous system is involved a fairly acute meningoencephalitis ensues, and this has been mistaken for tuberculous meningitis.

Clinical diagnosis

T. b. rhodesiense infection should be suspected in patients from endemic areas with prolonged febrile illness, jaundice, myocarditis or mental changes.

Treatment

Treatment is urgent and melarsoprol is the drug of choice used as described above for *T. b. gambiense* infections. The patients need prolonged follow-up. Diuretics and digoxin are given in cardiac failure. If melarsoprol fails to cure, nitrofurazone orally or diazoaminobenzene (Berenil) given by intramuscular injection may be used.

Laboratory identification of African trypanosomes

The trypomastigotes are usually identified in blood films or lymph node aspirates. When they are present in numbers too small to be recognized in normal smears, they may be found by concentration methods or by inoculation of blood or tissue fluids into laboratory animals.

T. b. rhodesiense and *T. b. gambiense* are morphologically indistinguishable in the human host, and are differentiated on medical grounds. The only stage

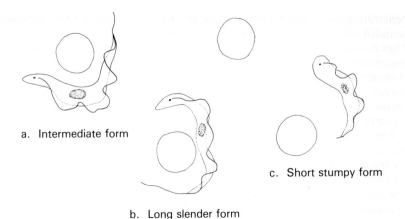

a. Intermediate form

c. Short stumpy form

b. Long slender form

Fig. 3.2   Pleomorphic African Trypanosomes, *T. b. rhodesiense* and *T. b. gambiense*, in blood.

occurring in man is the trypomastigote. The trypomastigotes are pleomorphic, and the blood contains forms differing in shape and size, in the presence or absence of a free flagellum and in other details. The undulating membrane is always well developed and conspicuous, the nucleus is central and the kineto-plast is small and subterminal. There may be three forms in the blood: the 'slender' form is long and thin, averaging 29 μm in length, with a long free flagellum; the 'stumpy' form is short and stout, averaging 18 μm in length, and is usually without a free flagellum; the 'intermediate' form averages 23 μm in length, and has a free flagellum of medium length (Fig. 3.2). The slender forms usually predominate, and the proportion of stumpy forms apparently increases as the host develops an immunity to the infection.

In old infections trypomastigotes are usually absent from the blood, but are present in the cerebrospinal fluid. The trypomastigotes in the cerebrospinal fluid have the same morphological appearance as those in the blood, and in both these sites dividing trypomastigotes may be found.

American trypanosomiasis

American trypanosomiasis, commonly called Chagas' disease, is caused by *Trypanosoma cruzi*. Chagas' disease occurs in Central America, Mexico and South America, especially in Brazil and Argentina. It causes disease in man, but there are many animal reservoirs (such as armadilloes, opossums, wood rats, dogs, cats and pigs) in which it causes no apparent disability. Trypanosomes morphologically indistinguishable from *T. cruzi* occur in monkeys in Asia and the Malayan Archipelago, and also in bats.

T. cruzi appears in the blood in the early stages of infection but it is hard to find when the disease becomes chronic. Dividing forms are not found in the blood, and this is one of the characteristics that separates this species from *T. b. gambiense* and *T. b. rhodesiense*. Division occurs, during periodic disap-pearance of the parasites from the blood, in foci in the deeper organs, especially in the heart muscles and the voluntary muscles. (Fig. 3.3). The trypanosomes penetrate into the cells of these organs, where they lose their flagella and become rounded amastigotes. These amastigotes multiply by repeated binary fission. They destroy the adjoining tissue as they increase in number, and form cyst-like agglomerations known as pseudocysts. The amastigotes then become elongated, produce a flagellum each, and become transformed into epimastigotes. The epimastigotes in turn multiply by repeated binary fission, and finally give rise to trypomastigotes that reappear in the blood. This cycle is repeated over and over.

The vectors are blood-sucking bugs of the Order Reduviidae. Both mature and immature stages of the bug are susceptible to infection, and develoment of the trypanosomes takes place in the alimentary tract. In the mid-gut of the bug the trypomastigotes are transformed into epimastigotes, which multiply rapidly and gradually spread to the rectum. The epimastigotes are transformed finally to metacyclic trypomastigotes that are similar to the blood forms but have a more slender body. The cycle in the bug takes 6–15 days.

Development in the bug is thus in the 'posterior station'. Transmission is contaminative (as opposed to inoculative in African trypanosomiasis). The infective metacyclic trypanosomes are deposited in faeces on the mucous membranes and skin of man. The bugs usually defaecate while feeding, but occasionally the whole bug may be crushed and the trypanosomes are rubbed into the abrasions. The metacyclic trypanosomes penetrate the mucous membranes of the eyes or mouth, or the skin, and enter the subcutaneous cells of the reticulo-endothelial system, where they produce a local lesion referred to as a 'Chagoma'. They become amastigotes, multiply rapidly, then produce flagella to form epimastigotes. These in turn divide by binary fission, and finally produce trypomastigotes that appear in the blood 4–20 days after infection. These trypomastigotes later pass to the internal organs and continue development as amastigotes as previously described. Trypomastigotes are present in the blood in appreciable numbers only in acute cases during the first 3 or 4 days, but after that their appearance is irregular and in progressively diminishing numbers.

The infection in animals such as the armadillo, the opossum and the wood rat is probably maintained by some 80 species of reduviid bugs, and occurs over a very much larger geographical area than does the human disease. The infection in man, which presumably originated from the animal reservoirs, is now maintained in small foci involving only the house, the people living in the house, the bugs living in the roof and the walls, and the intimate domestic animals such as cats and dogs. The bugs drop from the thatched roof or emerge from cracks in the mud walls at night, and take meals from persons or animals sleeping on the floor.

Medical aspects of American trypanosomiasis

Pathogenesis

Infection is frequently subclinical, subjects having serological evidence of infection and harbouring trypanosomes but having no clinical signs of disease. In some, no acute initial illness occurs and chronic Chagas' disease appears years later. In a minority there is an initial febrile lasting some weeks. Infective trypomastigotes invade macrophages in the dermis in the area of the bite, and a local inflammatory swelling is produced which later subsides spontaneously. After macrophage and tissue cell invasion the trypomastigotes convert to amastigotes through promastigote and epimastigote stages. Within the cells the amastigotes repeatedly subdivide for about 5 days, destroying the cell and producing a 'pseudocyst' — a shell of the cell that contained parasites. The pseudocyst ruptures, liberating some of its contents as trypomastigotes into the blood stream where they reinvade tissue cells. Residual amastigotes and cellular remains at the site of the pseudocyst induce focal inflammatory areas that may eventually leave permanent fibrotic damage. Blood-borne trypomastigotes invade striated, smooth and cardiac muscle cells, neuroglial cells and macrophages during the acute stage. The resultant febrile illness lasts 6–8 weeks, and may be complicated by acute meningoencephalitis, carditis and generalized lymphadenopathy. Most patients recover, but a proportion develop chronic disease later, and up to 10 per cent may die in the initial illness.

The pathogenesis of chronic Chagas' disease is not fully understood. Newly invaded cells with living parasites are rarely found in chronic disease. Some damage may be the result of the initial illness, but there is evidence of an autoimmune process in operation. Antibodies reacting with cardiac tissue and striated muscle are found in these patients. The myocardium shows patchy fibrosis, the heart is dilated sometimes with mural thrombi, and there may be an apical aneurysm of endocardium through damaged myocardium. Inflammation spreading from invaded muscle cells in the gut and heart damages local parasympathetic ganglia and fibres. This parasympathetic damage causes partial denervation of the oesophagus and colon leading to motility disturbance, difficulty in onward propulsion of contents, stasis and dilatation — the 'mega' syndromes of Chagas' disease.

Clinical picture

Acute Chagas' disease

The primary illness often occurs in childhood, the reduviid bugs biting the face during sleep. Infective trypanosomes are rubbed into the bite wound, conjunctiva or lips when the child scratches. A local subcutaneous oedematous swelling known as a chagoma appears within a few days. When it appears on the cheek or around the orbit, together with an enlarged preauricular lymph gland, the condition is called Romana's sign. The swelling subsides, but 1–2 weeks later an acute febrile illness begins lasting up to 8 weeks. Enlargement of the liver and spleen, generalized lymphadenopathy and a macular rash may appear. Usually the illness gradually subsides and the child recovers, but myocarditis and meningoencephalitis are serious complications.

Myocarditis presents with tachycardia, cardiac dilatation and failure, arrhythmias and sometimes pericardial effusion. The picture is similar to rheumatic carditis. In acute meningoencephalitis the child has increasing headache and may become drowsy or comatose and convulse. The mortality of acute carditis and encephalitis is high. Overall, 10 per cent may die during acute Chagas' disease.

Chronic Chagas' disease

This may appear after a latent interval of many years. The commonest manifestations are chronic cardiac damage, being found in up to 10 per cent of the rural population in some areas. Chronic right-sided cardiac failure, heart block, sudden cardiac death, arrhythmias and embolic phenomena from mural cardiac thrombi are the usual manifestations. Damage to conducting tissues of the heart is particularly common. Chagas' disease is a leading cause of cardiac pathology in endemic areas.

The mega syndromes are associated with particular strains or 'zymodemes' of *T. cruzi* from certain geographical areas. Mega-oesophagus causes dysphagia, regurgitation, wasting, and spill-over of oesophageal contents into the lungs with recurrent pulmonary infections. Mega-colon causes severe constipation with abdominal distension and pain, faecal impaction and even intestinal obstruction.

Congenital Chagas' disease is seen occasionally. Transmission by blood transfusion is a real danger. Donors should be serologically screened. Treatment of blood with gentian violet in a final concentration of 0.025 per cent for 24 hours destroys trypomastigotes.

Clinical diagnosis

The acute disease has to be distinguished from other febrile illnesses, acute rheumatic carditis and viral encephalitides. A history of a recent chagoma may be helpful. Chest X-rays, electrocardiograms and contrast radiography are needed in the investigation of chronic Chagas' disease.

Management

Specific treatment for Chagas' disease is unsatisfactory. Nifurtimox, a rather toxic nitrofurans drug, has been used at a dose of 8 mg/kg orally daily for 4 months. An alternative is benznidazole orally 5 mg/kg daily for 60 days. The strongest indication for chemotherapy is in the acute early stage. These drugs are probably of no value in chronic Chagas' disease.

In cardiac disease with complete heart block pacemakers have been inserted and antiarrhythmic drugs may be needed. Digoxin is of dubious benefit, and beta-blockers potentially dangerous. Myotomy at the oesophageal–gastric junction is used in mega-oesophagus. Disimpaction of faeces may be needed in mega-colon, and resection of affected portions of colon may be carried out, but the prognosis is poor.

Laboratory identification of American trypanosomes

T. cruzi occurs in man in two forms, the trypomastigote stage in the blood and the amastigote stage in the tissues. The trypomastigote appears in the blood in the early stages of infection but is hard to find when the disease becomes chronic. Xenodiagnosis, the feeding of 'clean' reduviid bugs on a suspected patient, may be used to isolate trypomastigotes when they are present in very small numbers. Serodiagnosis, using CFT and IFAT, is also of considerable value (see Chapter 11).

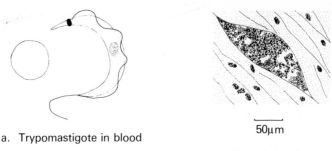

a. Trypomastigote in blood

50μm

b.   Amastigotes in
    section of muscle

Fig. 3.3 Monomorphic American Trypanosome, *T. cruzi.*

The trypomastigotes are monomorphic and medium-sized, about 20 μm in
length. The body is fairly thick with a pointed posterior end, and is often curved
in the form of a sickle or crescent. The nucleus is central and the kinetoplast is
sub-terminal. The kinetoplast is oval and relatively large so that it may cause the
body to bulge posteriorly. The undulating membrane is slightly developed,
being narrow and with only two or three convolutions, and a free flagellum is
always present (Fig. 3.3a). The parasites are not easy to find in stained preparations as they are fragile, and easily ruptured when the blood film is spread.
Dividing forms are not found in the blood.

Division occurs, during periodic disappearances of the parasites from the
blood, in foci in the deeper organs. The trypomastigotes penetrate into the cells
of these organs, where they lose their flagella, become rounded, and assume the
amastigote form. These amastigotes are usually spherical, about 1.5–4 μm in
diameter, but they are sometimes ovoid, about 5 × 3 μm. They multiply by binary
fission, destroy the adjoining tissues as they increase in numbers, and form cyst-
like agglomerations with no special wall derived either from the parasite or from
the host (Fig. 3.3b). Individual amastigotes may be seen in smear preparations,
or the pseudocysts may be recognized in histological sections of muscle.

Control of trypanosomiasis

Control of trypanosomiasis gambiense depends largely on active case detection
and treatment, and on the destruction of tsetse flies by application of insecticides such as Dieldrin to their breeding sites from the ground or the air. New
methods of control, using ultra-low-volume application of decamethrin and
other insecticides from fixed-wing aircraft or helicopters, have been developed.
Pentamidine, given by injection in one dose of 4 mg/kg intramuscularly, can
provide individual protection for about six months.

Trypanosomiasis rhodesiense is a zoonosis, and often affects hunters and
fishermen entering areas where there is infected game. Control is more difficult,
because elimination of the animal reservoir is impracticable as well as undesir-
able. Pentamidine cannot be used, so prevention depends largely on case
detection and treatment, and on tsetse control.

Control of American trypanosomiasis may ultimately depend on improvements in housing that eliminate domestic habitats of reduviid bugs, but this is costly. In the meantime control relies on spraying houses with residual insecticides such as hexachlorocyclohexane (HCH). Separation of households from reservoirs in domestic animals such as hens seems impracticable.

Further reading

Greenwood BM, Whittle HC. The pathogenesis of sleeping sickness. *Trans Roy Soc Tropical Med Hyg* 1980; **74**: 716–25.

Köberle F. Chagas' disease and Chagas' syndrome: the pathology of American trypanosomiasis. *Adv Parasitol* 1968; **6**: 63–116.

Lumsden WHR. The African trypanosomiases. *Br Med Bull*; 1970; **28**: 34–8.

Marsden PD. American trypanosomiasis: Chagas' disease. In: Weatherall DJ, Ledingham JGG Warrell DA (eds) *Oxford Textbook of Medicine*. Vol. 1. Oxford: Oxford University Press, 1983, 410–12.

Molyneux DH, Ashford RW. *The biology of Trypanosoma and Leishmania, parasites of man and domestic animals*. London: Taylor and Francis, 1983.

Mulligan HW, Potts WH (eds). *The African trypanosomiases*. London: Allen and Unwin, 1970.

WHO and FAO *The African trypanosomiases*. Geneva: WHO Technical Report Series No. 635, 1979.

4

Leishmania

The second genus of haemoflagellates that causes disease in man is *Leishmania*. The disease leishmaniasis occurs in Central and South America, China, India, Soviet Central Asia, the Middle East, Arabia, Africa and the Mediterranean area. *Leishmania* is parasitic in man, dogs, gerbils and other mammals, and the animals often act as reservoirs of the human infection. Leishmaniasis is transmitted by the sandflies *Lutzomyia* and *Phlebotomus*. It occurs in three forms, namely cutaneous leishmaniasis or 'oriental sore', mucocutaneous leishmaniasis or 'espundia', and visceral leishmaniasis or 'kala-azar'.

The genus *Leishmania*, like *Trypanosoma* discussed in Chapter 3, has two cycles of reproductive development, one in the human or animal host and one in the insect host. Unlike the trypanosomes, however, flagellate forms of *Leishmania* never occur in the vertebrate hosts, but only in the insect vectors or in culture. The forms found in human or vertebrate hosts are morphologically identical, and are small spherical or ovoid amastigote forms, incapable of translatory movement. In the insect vector the developmental stages are promastigote forms that are actively motile, and although they possess a flagellum they lack an undulating membrane at all stages of development — a characteristic which at once distinguishes them from the trypomastigote and epimastigote forms assumed by *Trypanosoma* in the insect host.

Until recently it was considered that the three types of leishmaniasis mentioned above were caused by infections with three different species of *Leishmania, L. tropica* producing cutaneous leishmaniasis, *L. braziliensis* producing mucocutaneous leishmaniasis, and *L. donovani* producing visceral leishmaniasis. These three species, morphologically indistinguishable in both the vertebrate host and the insect vector, were separated mainly on clinical characters. Recent work, however, has shown that this classification is an oversimplification. Although there are only three basic forms of leishmaniasis there are many variations within these forms, and the clinical picture and the epidemiology of the disease are different in different parts of the world. It is now accepted that the three types of disease are produced not by three single species but by three groups or complexes of species.

The species and sub-species of *Leishmania* are differentiated by a combination of clinical, pathological, serological, biochemical and geographical differences. Each geographical region appears to have its own particular combination of vector and type of disease. However, since the leishmanias are all transmitted by the same genera of sandflies and are morphologically indistinguishable under the ordinary light microscope, it is convenient to consider them together, to describe in detail the biology of one species complex, and then to consider how the other species differ.

Cutaneous leishmaniasis

Old World cutaneous leishmaniasis

The classical 'oriental sore', with its ulcerating lesion or lesions, is caused by infection with parasites of the *L. tropica* complex, namely *L. tropica* and *L. major* (although some workers refer to them as sub-species of *L. tropica*, namely *L. t. minor* and *L. t. major*). Infection is limited to local lesions of the skin and subcutaneous tissue, and the disease has various local names such as Aleppo button and Delhi boil. Oriental sore occurs in India, Africa, Arabia, the Middle East, Soviet Central Asia and the Mediterranean area. Parasites causing diffuse cutaneous leishmaniasis have been recorded from several parts of Africa, and one of these has been named *L. aethiopica*; their relationship with the *L. tropica* complex has not yet been elucidated.

The infective form of cutaneous leishmaniasis, which is introduced into the subcutaneous tissue by the biting sandfly, is the promastigote. It has a free flagellum as long as, or longer than, its body. The promastigotes either invade or else are ingested by the macrophages or endothelial phagocytes (histocytes or reticuloendothelial cells), and once inside the macrophages they lose their flagella and round up to assume the amastigote form. These multiply by binary fission until the cytoplasm of the macrophage becomes packed with them. Finally the cell distintegrates and releases the contained parasites, which then enter fresh macrophages to continue their multiplication. The initial lesion appears on the skin at the site of the bite in the form of a papule, from which the parasites can be recovered.

The incubation period during which the amastigotes are multiplying, before the development of the 'boil' or 'sore', usually lasts 2–3 months. When ulceration of the skin finally develops, the amastigotes are more or less confined to the deeper, and comparatively bacteria-free, tissues at the base of the ulcer; but they also occur in large numbers in the macrophages inhabiting the unbroken skin surrounding the ulcer.

It has been shown that mechanical transmission can be effected by biting flies of the genus *Stomoxys* (the stable fly), but in nature only sandflies of the genus *Phlebotomus* or *Lutzomyia* are known to be carriers, and these flies can only transmit the infection after the amastigotes have undergone a cycle of development in the gut of the fly. Sandflies feeding on the skin surrounding a tropical sore take up the amastigote parasites into the gut — they take up free amastigotes as well as those within the monocytes. In the sandfly the amastigote elongates and become spindle-shaped, the kinetoplast assumes a position at the anterior end, and a long free flagellum is given off. This is now the promastigote form, and is found only in the sandfly or in laboratory cultures. The early promastigotes are short, ovoid or pear-shaped bodies, 5–10 μm long by 2–3 μm wide; the fully developed ones are long and slender, measuring 10–15 μm long by 1–2 μm wide. The nucleus is central and the kinetoplast lies transversely near the anterior end (Fig. 4.1c).

The promastigotes multiply rapidly by longitudinal binary fission in the midgut of the sandfly, and an enormous number of flagellates is produced. These tend to spread forwards and accumulate in the anterior part of the insect's

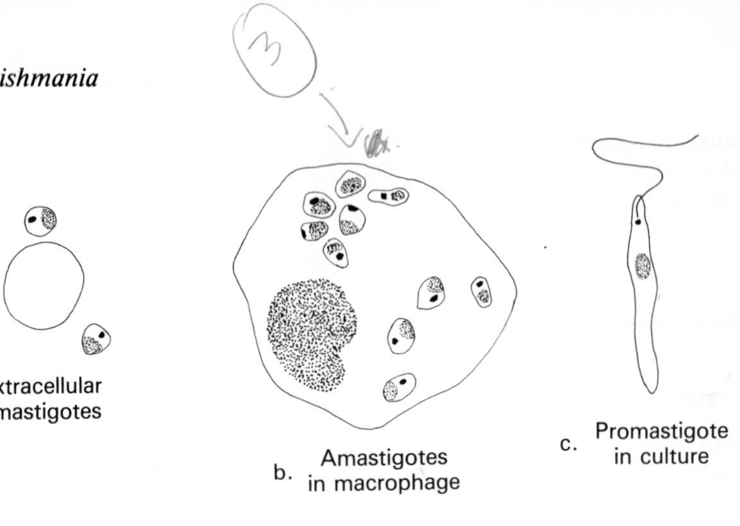

a. Extracellular
    amastigotes

b. Amastigotes
    in macrophage

c. Promastigote
    in culture

5μm

Fig. 4.1 Leishmania.

alimentary canal. By the end of the third day there are masses of them free in the proventriculus and pharynx, and also attached to the gut walls in these regions. By the end of the fifth day they occur in massive clusters, and by the end of the seventh day multiplication and invasion of the oesophagus and pharynx has proceeded so far that the passages of the gut become blocked. At this stage the fly is infective. When the sandfly tries to feed the parasites block the flow of blood, but some of the promastigotes are regurgitated, carried by the saliva to be deposited on the skin, and so cause a fresh infection. This is development in the 'anterior station' (see p. 59) even though infection is by contamination and not by inoculation. There may also be transmission when the bitten person rubs the sandfly into the abrasion while scratching the bite. Once they are in the skin the promastigotes enter, or are ingested by, macrophages, where they become transformed into amastigotes and develop as described above.

The disease produced is usually a mild condition, tending to self-cure with resulting immunity. As a rule there are no generalized symptoms. The sores are distributed on exposed parts of the body, particularly on the face and extremities. They are usually multiple, but may sometimes be single or limited to two or three. Human infections in some parts of Africa tend to be long-lasting and to produce a diffuse infection of the skin rather than ulcers. These infections are superficially similar to South American infections produced by some of the *L. mexicana* complex of parasites.

New World cutaneous leishmaniasis

Some of the parasites in the *L. braziliensis* and *L. mexicana* complexes may, especially in the early stages of the infection, cause typical 'oriental sores'. In the *L. mexicana* complex diffuse cutaneous leishmaniasis may also develop. However, while the parasites that cause oriental sores in the Old World remain restricted to the skin, those in the New World tend to invade the adjacent mucous membranes, either by direct spread or by metastasis through the lymphatics or blood stream. Secondary lesions may occur on the mucous membranes or on the skin, often after many years.

Medical aspects of cultaneous leishmaniasis

Pathogenesis

After the deposition of promastigotes by the sandfly, amastigote forms develop and subdivide within dermal macrophages which congregate and proliferate locally. A cell-mediated immunity infiltrate of lymphocytes localizes the infection and produces a nodule. Within a few weeks marked local inflammatory reactions against parasitic antigens and occlusion of local blood vessels by cellular pressure cause local necrosis and ulcer formation in the nodule. This results in a circular ulcer with a raised edge and some surrounding erythema. In some varieties lymphatic spread occurs to local lymph glands. Secondary bacterial infection is not uncommon. Healing is slow, taking several months, and a depressed scar remains. In some individuals the lesion fails to heal and gradually extends, resembling tuberculous lupus vulgaris. This condition is known as *leishmaniasis recidiva*, and is thought to be due to excessive T-cell hypersensitivity to parasite antigens.

In some people with cutaneous leishmaniasis in Ethiopia and Venezuela, cell-mediated immunity is deficient, and spreading infiltrated nodular lesions full of infected macrophages result. Lymphocyte reaction is lacking, and the condition is known as disseminated cutaneous leishmaniasis.

Clinical picture

The basic lesions are one or more nodules that break down after a few weeks to form indolent ulcers with raised edges. These ulcers are usually on areas of the skin liable to sandfly bites, such as the face and arms. The ulcers are not painful unless secondarily infected, and do not itch. Healing occurs slowly over 3–12 months. There are variations on this theme depending on the strain of parasite and the geographical location (see Table 4.1).

The incubation period varies from 2 weeks to several months.

Clinical diagnosis

The diagnosis must be considered in anybody from an endemic area with chronic skin ulcers. There are many other causes of chronic skin ulceration in tropical areas, including (1) phagedenic tropical ulcer which is necrotic and painful, (2) Buruli ulcer due to *Mycobacterium ulcerans*, which is painful and flattish with undermined edges, (3) guinea-worm ulcers, (4) malignant epitheliomas, (5) sickle cell disease causing ankle ulcers of an avascular nature, (6) primary yaws causing a proliferative lesion, and (7) tuberculous lupus vulgaris.

Table 4.1 Clinical characteristics of some varieties of cutaneous and mucocutaneous leishmaniasis

Organism	Distribution	Reservoir hosts	Remarks
L. tropica complex			
L. tropica	Mediterranean and North African coasts, Middle East, Southern Russia, West India, Pakistan	Man, dog	Urban; often facial and solitary; not severe
L. major	Middle East, North Africa and sub-Saharan Africa, Asia	Rodents	Rural; can be multiple, quite severe, sometimes local lymphadenopathy
L. aethiopica	Ethiopia, Kenya, South Yemen	Rock hyraxes	Mild; occasionally diffuse cutaneous leishmaniasis
L. mexicana complex			
L. m. mexicana	Mexico, Belize, Guatemala, Yucatan	Forest rodents	Chiclero's ulcers; single skin lesion on ear, face or hand
L. m. amazonensis	Amazon basin	Rodents and marsupials	Not severe; sometimes diffuse cutaneous leishmaniasis
L. braziliensis complex			
L. b. braziliensis	Brazil, Peru, Ecuador, Bolivia, Paraguay, Colombia	Forest rodents	Mucocutaneous leishmaniasis (see below)
L. b. peruviana	Western Peru	Dog	'Uta'; mild, on nose and lips

Treatment

Cutaneous leishmaniasis has a strong tendency towards self-healing. Most lesions will gradually improve if kept clean, covered, and free from bacterial infection by using local antiseptics, e.g. weak eusol. Infra-red treatment has been suggested as leishmania are sensitive to heat. In those with large ulcers or multiple ulcers sodium stibogluconate can be used as in visceral leishmaniasis — sometimes it is injected locally as well.

Disseminated cutaneous leishmaniasis responds poorly to chemotherapy. Sodium stibogluconate or amphotericin may induce remissions. *Leishmania recidiva* also responds poorly. Grenz rays, intralesional steroids and curettage may produce some improvement.

Mucocutaneous leishmaniasis

Mucocutaneous leishmaniasis, or 'espundia, is caused by *L. b. braziliensis*, and occurs in Central and South America. The first sign of infection is usually a slow-healing extensive oriental sore; and it is probable that the disfiguring disease of espundia is secondary, perhaps occurring long after the initial lesion has healed. The life-cycle and transmission of *L. braziliensis* is believed to be similar to those of other species; and dogs are thought to be reservoir hosts in parts of Brazil.

Espundia first appears as a papule that extends and finally ulcerates. The parasites occur in the macrophages infiltrating the dermis, and are localized in the reticuloendothelial cells of the margins and base of the lesions, and in the local lymph glands and lymphatics. The sores are usually single, but sometimes there are many. Espundia is a much more serious disease than cutaneous leishmaniasis because it can spread locally or metastasize by the lymphatics to the mouth and nose and cause extensive destruction and scarring of the oropharynx, hard palate, nose and even the larynx. Hideous deformity of the face results, and the victim may die of secondary sepsis or bronchopneumonia.

The incubation period varies from one week to several months. The infected individual may have some natural immunity, or immunity may be acquired following a naturally cured infection. Self inoculation, is sometimes practised to avoid facial scarring.

Medical aspects of mucocutaneous leishmaniasis

Treatment

Espundia should be treated with sodium stibogluconate as for visceral leishmaniasis (see below), or with amphotericin if this fails. Secondary sepsis needs antibiotic treatment.

Visceral leishmaniasis

Visceral leishmaniasis, or kala-azar, is caused by parasites of the *L. donovani* complex; there are differences of opinion as to whether this complex includes several species of *Leishmania* or several sub-species of the one species *L.*

donovani. Kala-azar occurs in China, Assam, India, Central Asia, Africa, the Mediterranean area and Central and South America.

The disease occurs in four main forms, which are clinically and epidemiologically distinct. These are:

1. Indian kala-azar, which occurs mainly in children and young adults. There is no evidence of any animal reservoir.
2. Mediterranean kala-azar, which occurs in children under the age of 5 years. There is a reservoir in dogs.
3. East African kala-azar, which occurs in children and young adults. This form frequently shows skin infections and mucocutaneous lesions. Wild mammals, but not dogs, act as reservoirs.
4. American kala-azar, which is similar to the Mediterranean form but not necessarily caused by the same parasite. Wild and domestic dogs act as reservoirs.

In the early stages of infection the parasites are confined to the skin, and in some cases there may be an identifiable papule or ulcer. Later the infected macrophages enter the blood stream and pass to the internal organs, where they invade the cells of the reticuloendothelial system and multiply intensively. Parasites are thus more abundant where there are numerous macrophages, as in the spleen, liver, intestinal mucosa, bone marrow and lymph glands.

Medical aspects of visceral leishmaniasis

Pathogenesis

Promastigotes that are deposited in the skin by sandflies are ingested by local macrophages, become amastigotes and repeatedly divide within the macrophages. As a result the macrophages rupture, and parasites.invade new macrophages which congregate locally and themselves, proliferate. In cutaneous leishmaniasis, and probably in most individuals infected with *L. donovani*, efficient cell-mediated immunity localizes the infection. In those who develop visceral leishmaniasis there is a specific defect in cell-mediated immunity against the parasite. When spread occurs by the blood stream the parasites invade macrophages in many parts of the body, including the spleen, liver and bone marrow, and in some geographical areas the lymph glands. In the spleen there is hyperplasia of macrophages and sinus endothelial cells, causing progressive splenic enlargement and hypersplenism with sequestration and destruction of cellular elements of the blood, resulting in anaemia and pancytopenia. Leucopenia increases liability to bacterial infections, thrombocytopenia may cause abnormal bleeding. Later, heavy infiltration of the marrow by infected macrophages interferes with blood cell production. The liver is enlarged with proliferation of Kupffer cells and infiltration with macrophages, lymphocytes and plasma cells. Liver function is maintained until late in the disease, when jaundice, hypoalbuminaemia and oedema may appear. Liver function usually returns to normal after treatment, but occasionally cirrhosis follows. Fever results from liberation of endogenous pyrogens by ruptured macrophages.

Immunity

Patients who contract visceral leishmaniasis have a specific defect in cell mediated immunity, and if untreated the disease is usually fatal in these individuals. The leishmanin intradermal test (the 'Montenegro' test), when positive, indicates a cell mediated immunity to leishmaniasis. In cases of visceral leishmaniasis the leishmanin test is negative during the disease but becomes positive after a cure. Many people in endemic areas show a positive leishmanin reaction although they give no history of visceral leishmaniasis. Subclinical infection, with spontaneous recovery, is probably commoner than clinical disease.

Clinical aspects

The incubation period is commonly 2–4 months, but periods ranging from 10 days to 9 years have been recorded. The onset is usually gradual. A local swelling at the site of the bite is sometimes seen in East Africa but not elsewhere. The first symptom is prolonged irregular fever with afebrile periods lasting some days. Classically there is a double daily rise in temperature, but this is not always seen. During the early febrile stages there is remarkably little constitutional upset, the appetite is maintained, but weight is lost.

As the disease progresses the spleen progressively enlarges, and discomfort is felt in the splenic area. Eventually, in untreated cases, the spleen becomes enormous, reaching the right iliac fossa. The liver also enlarges, but to a lesser extent. Generalized lymphadenopathy, particularly marked in the cervical region, is seen in India and also in the Sudan.

As the illness progresses further the patient becomes weakened, wasted and anaemic, and in lighter-skinned people the skin darkens. There is increased liability to bacterial infections such as pneumonia and dysentery. Diarrhoea is sometimes due to direct involvement of the gut by the leishmania. Jaundice, ascites and oedema may be seen in the late stages. Thrombocytopenia can result in abnormal bleeding tendencies. Proteinuria due to glomerular immune complex deposition is common; renal amyloidosis causing uraemia is also recorded.

Untreated visceral leishmaniasis is almost always fatal, running its course in 6–18 months. Intercurrent infection is a common cause of death. Sometimes the illness takes a fulminant course, the victim dying within a few weeks.

Post kala-azar dermal leishmaniasis (PKDL)

Some patients (about 10 per cent in India but fewer elsewhere) develop dermal lesions up to 5 years after apparently successful treatment. This is known as post kala-azar dermal leishmaniasis (PKDL), and consists of papular and macular lesions on the face and other parts of the body, sometimes including the mucous membrane of the mouth. The papules are full of dividing amastigotes, and they are an important source of sandfly infection, particularly in India where the disease is not a zoonosis. PKDL may be mistaken for leprosy. Visceral relapse does not occur, and PKDL normally responds to a further course of sodium stibogluconate.

Clinical diagnosis

During the early stages visceral leishmaniasis has to be distinguished from other chronic or relapsing febrile illnesses including tuberculosis, malaria and typhoid. With enlargement of the spleen, liver and sometimes lymph nodes, leukaemia, reticulosis and tropical splenomegaly need exclusion. The blood changes may simulate aplastic anaemia, but the clinical picture is different. Hyperglobulinaemia and the blood picture are suggestive of the diagnosis.

Treatment

Specific
Sodium stibogluconate is the best specific drug. It is given by daily intravenous injection in daily doses of 600 mg for an adult and 10 mg/kg for children; larger doses of 20 mg/kg daily have been used in Kenya. If intravenous injection is impracticable, the drug can be given intramuscularly. In Asia 6–10 daily injections may suffice, but in Kenya and the Sudan the parasite is more resistant and 30 daily injections or more may be needed. About 90 per cent respond to antimony, but the response rate may be considerably lower in Africa. An alternative drug is pentamidine 4 mg/kg in 4 ml of water intramuscularly daily for 10 days. Pentamidine is a toxic diamidine which may cause hypotension, liver damage and hypoglycaemia. If other drugs do not succeed, Amphotericin B, at a dose of 0.25–1 mg/kg by daily infusion for 4–8 weeks, can be tried. Recently rifampicin and isoniazid have been found to potentiate the action of pentostam in *L. mexicana amazonensis* infections.

Supportive
Treatment of complicating infections, blood transfusion, and a good diet are often required as well as specific therapy. Cases should be followed up to ensure that the infection is really cured. Splenectomy has occasionally been carried out in patients resistant to chemotherapy, and after splenectomy patients often respond to drug treatment.

Laboratory identification of leishmania

Flagellated forms of *Leishmania* do not occur in the vertebrate hosts, but only in the insect vectors or in cultures (see below). The forms found in man are the amastigotes; and those of the different types of leishmaniasis are morphologically indistinguishable, although they are found in different parts of the body in different infections. Amastigotes of cutaneous and mucocutaneous leishmaniasis occur in specimens obtained by aspiration from tissue at the edges of lesions in the skin or mucous membranes, and those of visceral leishmaniasis occur in biopsies of bone marrow, liver and spleen. The parasites may be found by microscopic examination of stained films or smears of this material.

These amastigote forms are similar to those of *T. cruzi*, being small, rounded or ovoid bodies, measuring about 2–4 μm along the largest axis, and incapable of translatory movement. The cell membrane is very delicate and can usually only be seen in fresh or heavily stained specimens. The nucleus is a solid-looking structure, round or oval, and usually situated either in the middle of the cell or along one side. The kinetoplast lies tangentially or radially to the nucleus, and may be rod-shaped or like a small dot. It is much smaller than the nucleus, and usually more heavily stained (Fig. 4.1a, b). A vacuole is often visible as a clear unstained space towards one end of the parasite. Sometimes, in a deeply stained film, some amastigotes will exhibit a fine red line running from the kinetoplast to the rim of the cell. This is the axoneme or rhizoplast, and is the base of the future flagellum (which only develops in the insect vector). The amastigote forms are commonly called Leishman–Donovan bodies, although strictly this name should be restricted to the amastigote of *L. donovani*.

The parasites, however, are usually present in smears only in small numbers, and as they are small and not motile they are difficult to identify. It has therefore become routine to culture some of the biopsied material in blood agar media, in which the amastigotes usually grow well and develop into large numbers of the active flagellated promastigotes which are relatively easy to recognize. The most widely employed culture technique uses the classical NNN medium, a blood agar medium with a liquid overlay: but there are now many specialized media for growing particular strains of *Leishmania*.

Frequently, in old infection, parasites are very scanty, and in these cases — and as a method of diagnosis in clinics — serological rests may provide useful confirmatory evidence. The method of choice is the Montenegro skin test (or the Leishmanin test) in which 0.1 ml of a suspension of dead promastigotes is inoculated intradermally. In positive cases an erythematous wheal develops after 48 hours. Other serological tests, including the IFAT and ELISA, are also available: they are of considerable value in confirming a tentative diagnosis, but specific antigens are not yet available.

Control

Sandflies are very susceptible to modern insecticides, and in areas where sandflies are endophilic, biting inside houses, spraying with insecticides as for malaria control has proved effective. The control of Indian visceral leishmaniasis is an example of this. Where the insects are exophilic, biting outside houses, and the disease is a zoonosis involving wild mammals, house spraying is ineffective.

In some places where there is a canine reservoir, identification and destruction of infected dogs has proved effective; but control of reservoirs in wild rodents is not usually feasible. Where humans are the main reservoir of the disease, as in Indian visceral leishmaniasis, case detection and treatment is very important. Control of cutaneous leishmaniasis is helped by the removal of rubble and refuse which provides breeding places for sandflies — and spraying of such breeding sites with residual insecticides has also proved valuable.

Prophylactic immunization with live cultures of *L. tropica* has been practised with success in the Middle East, and a new vaccine is at present being developed for the prevention of cutaneous leishmaniasis. Control has proved more difficult in South America, where new settlements in forest areas should be separated by cleared areas from the surrounding jungle.

Further reading

Manson-Bahr PEC, Apted FIC. (eds) *Manson's Tropical Diseases*, 18th edn. 93–115. London: Bailliere Tindall, 1982.

Molyneux DH, Ashford RW. *The biology of Trypanosoma and Leishmania, parasites of man and domestic animals*. London: Taylor and Francis, 1983.

Smith DH. Leishmaniasis. *Med Int* 1984; **2**: 154–60.

WHO The leishmaniases. Geneva: *W.H.O. Technical Report Series* 701, 1984.

Williams P, Coelho, M de V. Taxonomy and transmission of *Leishmania*. *Adv Parasitol* 1978; **16**: 1–42.

Part II
Helminthic infections

Medical parasitologists refer collectively to all parasitic worms as helminths, and the parasitic helminths of man are included in two groups, the Platyhelminthes (flatworms) and the Nematoda (roundworms). Platyhelminthes are dorsoventrally flattened, they have no body cavity, and the alimentary canal, if present, is blind-ending without an anus. Nematoda are rounded in cross-section, and have a body cavity and a straight gut with an anus. There are thousands of species of parasitic flatworms and roundworms, and many more thousands of species that are free-living.

The phylum Platyhelminthes includes two Classes, the Cestoidea or tapeworms and the Trematoda or flukes, both of which are composed of internal parasites of man and other animals. The tapeworm parasites of man are all found in the Subclass Cestoda. These are all hermaphrodite, and in none is there an intestine. The adult worms are found exclusively in the intestines of their hosts. Each tapeworm consists of a head with sucking organs and, in some species, an anterior disc-like extension called a rostellum, which may be armed with hooks. From this head stretches a long chain of segments, each with a complete set of male and female sexual organs, so that each tapeworm may in some ways be regarded as a colony of separate individuals. The flukes parasitic in man are all members of the Subclass Digenea. They are nearly all hermaphrodite, although in some the sexes are separate, and they possess a blind-ending alimentary canal that is usually shaped like an inverted letter Y. They occur in various organs of their hosts. Flukes are usually leaf-shaped, but some are cylindrical. They have no obvious head, the body is not segmented, and on the ventral surface of the body they have two suckers by means of which they are attached inside the host.

5
Tapeworms

Class Cestoda

The tapeworms that are parasitic in man in their adult form are all parasites of the small intestine. They have their anterior end modified to form the head or scolex, which is always provided with sucking organs. The suckers are usually rounded; but sometimes they are slit-like, and are then called bothria. Hooks are sometimes present on the head, carried on a terminal disc-like extension called the rostellum. The posterior part of the head is the proliferating area, which continuously buds off young segments. The undifferentiated segments form the neck, from which spring the differentiated segments or proglottids. The youngest and smallest segments are, of course, those nearest the neck, while the oldest and largest are furthest away. The segments furthest from the head each contain a uterus full of eggs, and are referred to as 'gravid'; those in the middle of the worm each have both male and female sexual organs and are referred to as 'mature'; while those nearest the neck either have no genitalia or have only the male genitalia, which develop before the female ones. So far as reproduction is concerned, each individual segment in itself constitutes a complete animal.

The entire 'colony' of segments is called a strobila, and varies in length in different species from a few millimetres to several metres. The shape of the segments varies not only in different species, but also according to the age of the segment. However, it is nearly always flattened, and the surface nearest to which the ovary lies is termed the ventral surface. The whole surface is covered by the tegument through which the animal absorbs its nourishment. Beneath the tegument the body consists of parenchyma, divided into cortical and medullary portions by a layer of longitudinal and transverse muscle fibres. The cortical parenchyma contains a large number of 'calcareous corpuscles', about 5–25 μm in diameter, which give the worm its white colour. These corpuscles have a complicated organic chemical structure, and contain calcium. The medullary parenchyma contains the excretory, nervous and reproductive systems; there is no alimentary canal. Excretion is by means of flame cells connected to longitudinal excretory canals which run through all the segments and discharge from the last segment. The nervous system consists of a ring of nerve fibres and ganglionic cells situated in the scolex, from which run a pair of main longitudinal nerve fibres. The remainder of the medullary parenchyma is filled by the reproductive organs. All medically important tapeworms are hermaphrodites, and the arrangement of the reproductive organs is important because it helps to differentiate the various types of tapeworms.

The male genitalia always develop before the female genitalia, and the plan on which they are arranged is the same in all the Cestoda. The testes are usually very numerous, although in the genus *Hymenolepis* there are only three testes. The testes are distributed throughout the segment, and from each testis arises a minute tubular vas efferens. The vasa efferentia unite to form a common duct, the vas deferens, the terminal portion of which is called the cirrus and is surrounded by a muscular organ called the cirrus sac. The cirrus sac is often small, but in *Hymenolepis nana* it is conspicuous and extends half-way across the segment. The cirrus sac is concerned with the protrusion of the cirrus, which is the male copulatory organ. Because the male and female organs mature at different times in the same strobila, a dilatation known as the seminal vesicle is developed on the vas deferens for storing the sperm. The cirrus sac opens into the genital atrium, which opens to the exterior by the genital pore; this is generally situated on the lateral margin of the segment but in some species is on the ventral surface. In some species there are two lateral genital pores per segment, one on each margin.

The major female reproductive organ is the ovary, usually bilobed, which discharges eggs into a minute oviduct. The oviduct divides into two larger ducts, one of which is called the vagina and leads directly to the genital atrium so that its opening is in the same cavity as the male cirrus. The other duct is called the uterus, and it later becomes filled with eggs. In the majority of human tapeworms the uterus is a blind-ending sac, but in some species (such as *Diphyllobothrium latum*) it opens to the exterior. The vagina often has a dilatation, the seminal receptacle, in which the sperms are stored. The oviduct also often shows a swelling known as the ootype, into which open the ovaries, the uterus, and the vitelline glands that supply the yolk cells. Surrounding, or opening into, the ootype is a gland called Mehlis' gland, often called the shell gland although

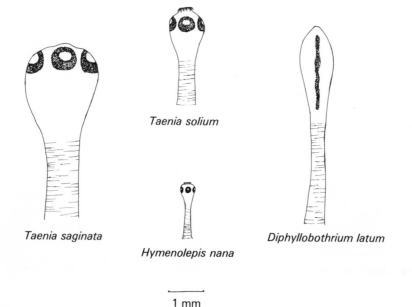

Taenia solium

Taenia saginata

Hymenolepis nana

Diphyllobothrium latum

1 mm

Fig. 5.1 Heads of tapeworms parasitic in Man.

probably it has nothing to do with the formation of the egg shell.

Fertilization occurs when spermatozoa are transferred to the vagina by means of the cirrus. Ova in one segment may be fertilized by the spermatozoa from the same segment, from another segment, or even from another worm. The ovum is fertilized in the ootype, and then receives the secretions from the vitelline gland and Mehlis' gland. It finally enters the uterus enclosed in the egg shell.

The Class Cestoda is divided into various Orders, two of which are of medical importance. These are Cyclophyllidea, in which the head is armed with four suckers and may or may not possess hooks (Fig. 5.1), and the segments have one or two marginal genital pores (Fig. 5.2); and Pseudophyllidea, in which the head is armed with two sucking grooves (bothria) and no hook (Fig. 5.1), and the segments have single genital pores on the flat ventral surface (Fig. 5.2).

In the Pseudophyllidea there is only one species that commonly parasitizes man. In the Cyclophyllidea there are at least two families, the Taeniidae and Hymenolepididea, which are of medical importance. Of these, the family Taeniidae is the more important.

Family Taeniidae

These are usually large tapeworms and the head, when armed, shows a double row of hooks. The hooks have a common shape in all members of the family. In the family are two genera of medical importance, *Taenia* and *Echinococcus*. The genus *Taenia* has the characteristics of the family, and the genus *Echinococcus* can be distinguished from *Taenia* by its small size (about 4 mm), by the fact that it has only 3–5 segments, and by the uterus which lacks the characteristic branching of the *Taenia* uterus.

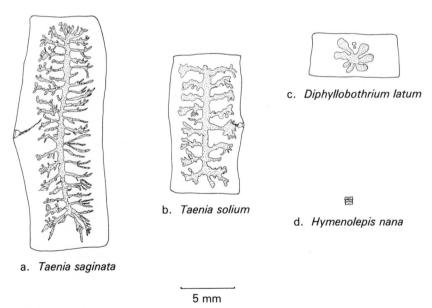

c. *Diphyllobothrium latum*

b. *Taenia solium*

d. *Hymenolepis nana*

a. *Taenia saginata*

5 mm

Fig. 5.2 Gravid segments of tapeworms found in Man.

T. solium and *T. saginata*

In the genus *Taenia* are many species affecting man and animals. Two of these species. *T. solium* and *T. saginata*, are relatively common and occur in their adult forms in the small intestine of man. They are easily differentiated. *T. solium* is usually 2–3 m long, but may be as long as 5 m, and is composed of up to 900 segments. The head is globular with a diameter of about 1 mm, and has a rostellum which bears a double crown of about 28 hooks (Fig. 5.1). The uterus in the gravid segment has up to 12 lateral branches (Fig. 5.2). *T. saginata* measures 3–4 m in length, but may be as long as 10 m, and is composed of over 1000 segments. The head is 1.5 mm in diameter and has neither rostellum nor hooks (Fig. 5.1). The uterus in the gravid segment has more than 15 lateral branches (Fig. 5.2).

Life-history of *T. solium* and *T. saginata*

It is convenient to start with the fertilized eggs in the gravid uterus. The shape, size and colour of the eggs, and the appearance of the embryo, vary considerably in different species of cestodes — but the eggs of all species of Cyclophyllidea have the same general structure. The egg, as originally formed in the oviduct, consists of an embryo with six hooks (a 'hexacanth embryo' or 'oncosphere') surrounded by a wall known as an embryophore. This in turn is surrounded by a layer of yolk cells, and outside the yolk layer is an outer egg shell. Some cestode eggs are colourless (e.g. *Hymenolepis*), others are straw-coloured or light yellow (e.g. *Diphyllobothrium*), while those of all species of *Taenia* are brown.

The eggs of any species of tapeworm (indeed of any helminth) vary in size and shape within fairly wide limits. The embryo of *T. solium* or *T. saginata* is surrounded by a thick striated embryophore about 35 μm in diameter. The outer egg shell is a very delicate covering, and this, together with the yolk cells, is usually lost during the passage of the egg out of the segment so that the 'egg', when passed, consists only of the embryo and the embryophore (Fig. 9.2). The last segments of *Taenia* consist simply of a muscular wall containing the uterine sac full of eggs (Fig. 5.2). The uterus in these gravid segments consists of a central stem with a number of compound lateral branches on each side — although in some Taeniids (e.g. *Echinococcus*) it may be sacculated.

As the uterus of *Taenia* does not open on the surface of the segment, the eggs can only escape into the lumen of the gut by the rupture of the segment, which may occur when the segment becomes detached from its neighbours and passes out with the faeces. The majority of the eggs pass out in the unruptured segment, but sometimes the segment disintegrates before it is passed. Not uncommonly the segments actively make their escape through the anus and so reach the ground, or become entangled in the patient's underclothes.

No further development of the hexacanth embryo can take place until it has been swallowed by a suitable host. It is not known how long the eggs may remain viable, but it has been shown that they can survive for 6 months in flooded pasture land. In species of cestodes occurring in the family Taeniidae the larval stage is completed in a vertebrate intermediate host, but in other cestodes it may occur in an invertebrate host (e.g. *Dipylidium caninum* in fleas), or it may

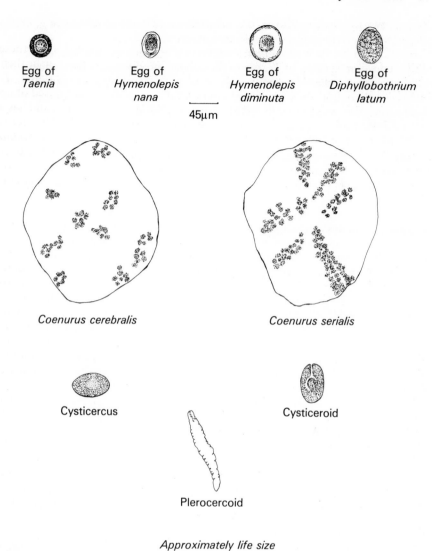

Egg of
Taenia

Egg of
*Hymenolepis
nana*

45µm

Egg of
*Hymenolepis
diminuta*

Egg of
*Diphyllobothrium
latum*

Coenurus cerebralis

Coenurus serialis

Cysticercus

Cysticeroid

Plerocercoid

Approximately life size

Fig. 5.3 Immature stages of Cestodes. The hydatid cyst is not illustrated because of its very large size.

require two intermediate hosts, one invertebrate and one vertebrate (e.g. *Diphyllobothrium latum* in *Cyclops* and freshwater fishes).

In *T. saginata* the normal intermediate host is a bovine, and the larval stage cannot develop in man. In *T. solium* the normal intermediate host is the pig, but the larva can also develop in man. It follows that autoinfection in man can occur with *T. solium* but not with *T. saginata*. Adult tapeworms are comparatively innocuous, but infection with larval stages may cause serious symptoms — and *T. solium* is therefore a potentially dangerous parasite.

When the egg of *T. solium* or *T. saginata* is swallowed by a suitable host, the hexacanth embryo escapes from the embryophore, probably in the duodenum or jejunum, and by means of its hooklets bores into the mucous membrane and eventually reaches a lymph space or blood vessel. The embryo is then carried by the blood to some part of the host's body, where it develops to form a larva known as a cysticercus. The cysticercus is a small fluid-filled bladder that contains a single scolex similar to that of the adult worm (Fig. 5.3). The larval form of *T. saginata* is known as *Cysticercus bovis* and that of *T. solium* as *Cysticercus cellulosae*. The development of *C. bovis* and *C. cellulosae* is similar.

Probably the majority of the embryos perish as a result of being carried by the blood or lymph to unsuitable sites, but those that reach subcutaneous or intermuscular connective tissue undergo further development. The first stage of this new development is a breaking down and liquefaction of the contents of the embryo at its centre. The embryonic hooks persist for some time, but having served their purpose they eventually disappear leaving a smooth double-walled bladder. A dimple now appears on the surface of this bladder, and this gradually invaginates. At the bottom of the invagination the head of the future tapeworm begins to develop, complete with suckers. When seen in muscle the bladder is surrounded by a resistant fibrous sheath, which must be stripped off to reveal the larva underneath. This sheath is not formed by the cysticercus, but is a result of reaction by the mammalian host. The cysticercus takes 2–3 months to develop fully.

The larva remains in this encysted state until swallowed by man in insufficiently cooked meat. When this occurs, the fibrous capsule is dissolved in the small intestine and the head evaginates from the cyst and attaches itself to the host's gut wall by its suckers. The bladder is then absorbed, and the neck begins to bud off the proglottides which, when fertilized and gravid, will appear in the faeces some 2–3 months later.

It is important to realize that, since man is the only host for the adult forms of *T. solium* and *T. saginata*, the respective larval infections in porcine and bovine animals are always from a human source, and due to some failure in sanitation.

T. saginata has a world-wide distribution, but tends to be particularly common among races who prefer their beef in an undercooked or even raw state. The larval form, *C. bovis*, normally develops in the muscles of the jaw, heart, diaphragm or shoulder of cattle, though other sites have been recorded; sometimes the oesophagus is invaded and may be the only site involved. The cysticercus, when fully developed (after 3–6 months), measures about 8 × 5 mm. Cysticerci can survive in muscle for 6–9 months, but eventually they die and become calcified.

Taenia solium, like *T. saginata*, has a world-wide distribution, but the infection is confined to people who eat pork. Unlike the larva of *T. saginata*, however, the larval form of *T. solium* develops a man as well as in the pig; but whereas the larval form (*C. cellulosae*) in its normal host (the pig) seems to produce no symptoms, grave illness is often caused by its presence in man — hence the medical importance of the infection. When the egg of *T. solium* is swallowed by the pig, further development takes place usually in the tongue, foreleg, thigh and neck. The cysticerci may live in the pig for several years, but they finally die and become calcified. In man the severity of the signs and symptoms is dependent on the number of cysticerci and their location in the body.

The cysticercus becomes fully developed in about 10 weeks, but its presence as a tiny white pin-head-sized body can be detected by the naked eye a fortnight after it has settled down in the tissue. The development of the cysticercus is similar to that of *C. bovis*. It has a milky-white bladder, which tends to be larger than that of *C. bovis* and may be as large as 10–15 mm. It can be distinguished from *C. bovis* by the fact that the scolex, which shows up a small dark patch in the bladder, is armed with hooks. Man acquires the infection only by eating undercooked pork, and the pig is only infected by swallowing the eggs passed in the faeces of man.

Medical aspects of *T. saginata* infections

Clinical

Infections are usually asymptomatic, and their presence is first suspected when tapeworm segments are seen in the stools or when the segments wriggle through the anus causing discomfort and embarrassment. Abdominal discomfort and pruritus ani can be caused by this parasite. Other symptoms described are hunger pains, excessive appetite and diarrhoea, but these are uncommon, as also are episodes when tapeworm segments obstruct the appendix, pancreatic or common bile duct causing inflammation in these organs. Intestinal obstruction due to multiple worm infection is rare. Many of the symptoms that have been described only appear when the subject realizes that he is infected.

Treatment

Four 0.5 g tablets of niclosamide are chewed and swallowed with a glass of water after an overnight fast. The worm disintegrates in the intestine, but cure cannot be immediately guaranteed as the scolex is not seen in the stools. The stools should be examined for the reappearance of ova or segments 3 months and 6 months later. Children weighing 35 kg or more are given 1.5 g of niclosamide, those weighing 10–34 kg are given 1 g. An alternative treatment is paromomycin 1 g orally every 15 minutes for 1 hour.

Medical aspects of *T. solium* infections

Pathogenesis and clinical manifestations

Infection with the adult worm produces similar symptoms to those caused by *T. saginata*, although the detached segments are less lively and are unlikely to crawl through the anus. Infection with the larvae, cysticercosis, is serious. The larvae metastasize to many sites including skeletal muscle, brain, subcutaneous tissue, the myocardium and the eye. Cysts may remain alive for some years, and after death they are surrounded by an inflammatory reaction and eventually calcify. Many patients with cysticercosis have no symptoms, and the infection is dis- covered accidentally after radiology has shown calcified cysts in the muscles. However, cerebral cysticerci are dangerous, causing epilepsy (particularly common in South America and South Africa) and sometimes death in status epi- lepticus. Cysts in the central nervous system can cause a chronic encephalopathy with dementia, focal signs or internal hydrocephalus due to blocking of the aqueduct of Sylvius. Cerebral tumour may be mimicked. Cysts behind the retina can cause retinal detachment, uveitis, retinitis and sometimes blindness. Multiple myocardial cysts lead to cardiac failure, conduction defects or arrhyth- mias. Muscle involvement usually causes no symptoms, but massive invasion may cause muscle pains. Subcutaneous cysts are palpable and their nature is diagnosed after biopsy.

Clinical diagnosis

Cysticercosis should be considered as a cause of neurological and ophthalmic disease in endemic areas. Cysts do not calcify for some years, so will not be seen radiologically in the early stages, but serology will be positive (see Chapter 11). Computerized axial tomography and radio-isotope scans of the brain show multiple small lesions. Biopsy of palpable subcutaneous nodules may be diagnostic.

Treatment

Infection with the adult worm is treated with niclosamide as for *T. saginata*. Treatment should be preceded by an antiemetic (metaclopramide or prochlor- perazine) and followed by a saline purge 2 hours after dosing. This is to prevent regurgitation of ova into the stomach, hatching of ova in the intestine and sub- sequent cysticercosis. Exposure of ova to gastric juice is a prerequisite for hatch- ing of ova in the intestine.

   Until recently there has been no effective specific drug treatment for cysti- cercosis, but praziquantel (usually given with prednisone) gives promise of being useful in cerebral cysticercosis. Surgery of cerebral lesions is rarely helpful and is sometimes dangerous. Anticonvulsants are given to control epilepsy. Surgery and photocoagulation are used to treat retinal lesions.

Echinococcus granulosus

The second genus of medical importance in the Taeniidae is *Echinococcus*. The adult form of *Echinococcus* does not parasitize man; *Echinococcus* occurs in man only in the larval stage.

The adult worm, which has a world-wide distribution, usually occurs in the upper part of the small intestine of the domestic dog, but it may occur in many of the carnivores. Unlike *T. solium* and *T. saginata*, the adult is incapable of developing in the human host.

E. granulosus is the smallest tapeworm of domestic animals, measuring only 3–9 mm in length. It is remarkable not only for its small size, but for the fact that when fully grown it has only 3 or 4 (very rarely 5) segments, of which only the last one is gravid. The scolex is armed with two rows of hooks, about 30–36 in number, arranged in a circlet with large and small hooks alternating. The hooks have the characteristic form common to all members of the family Taeniidae. Four unarmed suckers are present on the scolex. The uterus in the gravid segments is seldom multilobed, as in *Taenia*, but is usually sac-like.

Unless the adult tapeworm occurs in very large numbers it appears to be quite harmless to its host, so that infections in the dog are usually only recognized by diligent search of the faeces, or else by examining the gut *post mortem*. This harmlessness of the adult tapeworm is in marked contrast to the pathogenicity of the larval stages, which occur in man and various herbivorous farm animals.

In spite of the small size of the adult worm, the eggs are the same size as those of the *Taenias*, and are in fact indistinguishable morphologically from *Taenia* eggs. *Echinococcus* eggs are very resistant to all normal conditions, and to many abnormal conditions. The eggs gain access to water or vegetation polluted by the faeces of infected dogs, and thence may be ingested by herbivorous animals. It is, however, important to remember that the dried proglottides containing the eggs often become attached to the hairs of dogs, and it appears likely that the great majority of human infections are acquired as a result of handling dogs whose coats have thus become infected. Such infections are probably acquired mainly by children, while adults are probably more usually infected by ingesting vegetables that have become contaminated by dog faeces.

The larval stage is known as a hydatid cyst. The eggs pass out of the dog's intestine with the faeces, either contained in the proglottides or free, and further development can take place in a variety of hosts. The optimum host is usually considered to be the sheep, but development can also take place in man, cattle, goats, pigs, horses, rabbits, and various other animals. In many of these animals, however, the cysts produced tend to be 'sterile' (i.e. no scoleces are developed). In horses nearly all the cysts are fertile, in sheep almost 90 per cent are fertile and in pigs almost 80 per cent. In cattle only about 10 per cent are fertile.

The hydatid cysts develop in various organs. The commonest site of infection is in the liver (60 per cent of infections) but the lungs, kidneys, spleen, omentum, heart, and not uncommonly the brain, may also be infected. Infection may even take place in the bone marrow, but here the cysts are generally sterile.

As in the *Taenias*, when the egg is swallowed the embryophore is digested and the hexacanth embryo escapes. By means of its hooklets it moves actively into the thickness of the digestive mucosa until it enters a blood vessel, where it is carried passively by the blood until it is held up by the narrowing capillaries. This filtering action of the capillaries probably explains the frequency of the hydatid in the liver and lungs. Once the embryo has reached a site of development, which it can do within 3 hours of being swallowed, it is exposed to attack by leucocytes and may be destroyed. However, a proportion of the embryos survive and develop slowly into hydatid cysts.

The hydatid cyst is developed from a single hexacanth embryo, but instead of the resultant bladder ceasing to develop when it has reached the size of about a centimetre, as happens in *T. solium* and *T. saginata*, it continues to expand to an indefinite extent, while the inner layer, instead of producing a single head or scolex, may produce many thousands of 'brood capsules' each containing 10–15 protoscoleces that can develop into adult tapeworms.

The bladder is normally spherical in shape, but its form depends on the organ in which it is growing because it is moulded by any resistant tissues, for instance in the liver by the bile ducts. No matter what its size, and it may be as large as a child's head, it is always filled with fluid. And as with *Taenia*, the origin of this fluid is in the liquefaction of the oncosphere.

The wall of the vesicle is thick and white, and is composed of two layers, an outer thick laminated layer and an inner thin plasmodial nucleated layer, called the germinal layer. There is another thick outer layer, the adventitious layer, which is independent of the parasite and is a protective capsule produced by the host and continued without any definite line of demarcation into the host's substance.

The germinal layer appears to serve three purposes: to lay down the laminated layer, which is 1–2 mm thick and which protects and supports the delicate contents of the cyst; to produce the fluid which fills the cyst cavity and which acts as a buffer and nutritive medium; and to give rise to the so-called brood capsules which in their turn give rise to the scoleces.

The head of the future tapeworm, the scolex, forms as a thickening of the inner wall of the brood capsule. This thickening rapidly develops into a small stalked bud, on which are formed the suckers and later the hooks, while inside it are often found the calcareous corpuscles that sometimes occur in the parenchyma of cestodes. As the scolex develops the hooks are gradually drawn down and retracted within the scolex, a manoeuvre apparently intended for the protection of the hooks, which come to lie below the suckers with their free ends opening forwards. The budding of scoleces in the brood capsule occurs at various times on different areas, and it eventually results in the production of some 10–15 scoleces in each brood capsule.

The pedicle attaching the brood capsule to the parent cyst is very delicate, and slight trauma may rupture it. When this happens, the brood capsule becomes detached and slowly sinks to the floor of the hydatid cyst, which eventually becomes carpeted with large numbers of these brood capsules and their released scoleces. The sediment so formed is known as 'hydatid sand', and in addition to recognizable brood capsules and scoleces it contains the resistant hooks and calcareous corpuscles from dead and disintegrated scoleces. Occasionally the germinal layer gives rise to cysts that are miniatures of the parent cyst, and which are referred to as 'daughter cysts'. These daughter cysts are complete with a laminated layer, germinal layer, and brood capsules, and are usually found lying free in the fluid of the parent cyst. They are apparently formed by pieces of germinal layer which may have become detached for one of a variety of reasons. The course of their formation is not known with certainty, but there is evidence that they are produced whenever circumstances occur that endanger the normal life of the cyst. For example, they tend to arise after trauma or after the entry of blood or bile or bacteria into the contents of the cyst. They occur not uncommonly in human infections, but are seen much less commonly in hydatids occurring in sheep or other susceptible animals.

The hydatid cyst is usually globular, but it adapts itself to the form of any resistant anatomical structure that it may encounter during its growth. Sometimes this results in herniation of both layers through some weak point in the surrounding adventitia. This hernia is known as an 'exogenous daughter cyst', and may finally sever all connection with the parent and from then on lead an independent existence.

Normally the infection is confined within the substance of the parent cyst, or of the exogenous daughter cysts, but sometimes trauma or surgical operation results in releasing the contents of the cyst. When such an accident occurs, the scoleces or pieces of germinal layer that have escaped into the peritoneal cavity may give rise to new cysts. A frequent sequel to the rupture of a hydatid cyst thus is the formation of multiple cysts. Multiple cysts so formed are often encountered, for example, in the peritoneum, and puncturing of hydatid cysts *in situ* may be very dangerous.

Echinococcus multilocularis

The main difference between this species and *E. granulosus* is that in *E. multilocularis* the hydatid cyst does not become encapsulated, but tends to spread like an invasive tumour.

The adult is not found in man, but is a parasite of foxes and wolves, and rarely of cats and dogs. The adult worms are embedded in the mucous membrane of the small intestine, as is *E. granulosus*. The adults differ only slightly from *E. granulosus*, in that they are slightly smaller, there are no lateral diverticula in the uterus, and the genital pore is situated anteriorly.

The eggs are indistinguishable from of those *E. granulosus*. They are infective to small rodents, such as field mice and voles, and to man. The hydatid cysts occur in the liver in most cases (over 90 per cent). They do not become encapsulated, and small vesicles of brood capsules, like miniature bunches of grapes, tend to infiltrate the surrounding liver substance and even pass to other organs like a malignant tumour. These spreading malignant cysts are known as 'multilocular' or 'alveolar' hydatids. This infection is focally distributed in certain countries or districts, and tends to be absent from others in which the ordinary form of hydatid is common.

Medical aspects of Echinococcus infections

Pathogenesis

Hydatid cysts produced by *E. granulosus* behave like slowly growing 'benign' tumours producing effects by local pressure. The diameter of the cysts increases by 0.25–1 cm per year, so that noticeable effects may not be found for 10 years in the liver. The liver is involved in about 60 per cent of cases, the lung in 25–40 per cent, and the brain, bones, kidney and spleen much less frequently. Expansion of cysts in these organs causes pain, blockage of tubes (e.g. bile ducts), and within the skull raised intracranial pressure. Rupture of a cyst occurs in about 10 per cent of cases, releasing highly allergenic fluid into body cavities, ducts and sometimes blood vessels. Systemic hypersensitivity reactions result. In minor leakages urticaria ensues, but serious anaphylactic shock may result and cause hypotension, bronchoconstriction, facial oedema and occasionally death. Infective protoscoleces are dispersed into the peritoneal cavity, biliary passages, pleura, bronchi or renal pelvis with establishment of many new cysts. Bacterial infection may follow rupture into bile ducts and bronchi. Solid hydatid growths in bone marrow cause pathological fractures.

Cysts caused by *E. multilocularis* behave like malignant tumours, causing local infiltration, tissue destruction and metastases.

Clinical picture

The clinical picture depends on the site and number of cysts, their rate of growth, and the duration of infection. Cysts take several years to reach a significant size; in the liver cysts may die, become surrounded by a thick fibrous capsule, and only be discovered at autopsy. Hepatic cysts present with local pain and a mass is felt projecting from the liver edge. Less commonly mild jaundice due to bile duct obstruction is found. If a cyst ruptures the peritoneum, bile passages or pleural cavity may be flooded with cyst fluid — urticaria, bronchoconstriction and vascular collapse following. Rupture into biliary passages can mimic cholecystitis.

Hydatid cysts in the lungs may be asymptomatic and discovered on chest X-ray, appearing as solid round shadows. Symptoms include cough, haemoptysis and chest pain, sometimes pleuritic in type. If rupture into the bronchial tree occurs there is a gush of watery fluid into the mouth, haemoptysis and a systemic hypersensitivity reaction.

In long bones cysts usually present with pathological fracture, and less commonly with bone pain. Intracranial cysts cause manifestations of raised intracranial pressure, generalized or focal fits and focal signs such as hemiplegia. Renal cysts cause loin pain and haematuria. Splenic cysts may push up the left diaphragm and rupture into the pleura. Multiple hydatid cysts in the peritoneum produce a distended tender abdomen, sometimes mistaken for tuberculous peritonitis.

E. multilocularis cysts in the liver grow more rapidly and resemble carcinoma of the liver in symptomatology and prognosis. Wasting, jaundice, local pain and an irregular hepatic mass are found.

Clinical diagnosis

In endemic areas suspicion of slowly growing tumours in liver, bones or kidneys should lead to consideration of hydatid disease, and prompt the performance of serological tests, e.g. complement fixation tests. The Casoni intradermal test is sensitive but not specific. Eosinophilia is sometimes present.

Radiologically liver cysts may show surrounding calcification. Liver scan or ultrasound are useful in diagnosis. In bones the X-ray shows osteolysis with or without a fracture. In the lungs the lesions may resemble tumours or abscesses. Sometimes the diagnosis is made during an exploratory operation. Blind needling is dangerous, as leakage of fluid causes anaphylaxis.

Treatment

Chemotherapy has proved disappointing. Mebendazole in large doses (30 mg/kg per day) for several months occasionally causes some shrinkage of hepatic cysts. Albendazole at a dosage of 5 mg/kg twice daily for several weeks is perhaps more promising and is under investigation.

Surgery is usually indicated, and cysts of *E. granulosus* can often be cleanly dissected from surrounding tissue because of encapsulation. Before attempted cyst removal the fluid contents should be aspirated and 10 ml of 10 per cent formalin or 1 per cent iodine instilled and left for 10 minutes to ensure that the contents are non infective in case of spillage. Anaphylactic shock is treated with intramuscular adrenaline 1/1000, hydrocortisone IV and infusion of volume expanders.

Treatment of *E. multilocularis* by surgery is more difficult, and often removal is incomplete or impossible so that recurrence is common. Mebendazole has been used with some temporary effect.

Dipylidium caninum

Another member of the family Taeniidae which occasionally parasitizes man in the adult stage is *Dipylidium caninum*. It is cosmopolitan in distribution, and the adult is normally found in the small intestine of dogs and cats. It is, however, occasionally found in children.

The adult worm measures 10–50 cm in length. The head is a rhomboid and bears four suckers and a retractile rostellum armed with several rows of small hooks. The mature segments are longer than they are broad, and have a genital pore on each margin. The eggs are like those of *Taenia*, but are slightly reddish in colour. The gravid proglottis appears reticulated owing to the presence of numerous uterine pockets each enclosing a packet of about 12 eggs enclosed in a membrane. The hexacanth embryos are about 34 μm in diameter.

The egg is swallowed by the larval stages of fleas. The oncosphere hatches in the gut and migrates to the haemocoele, where it becomes a cysticercoid. If a flea containing a cysticercoid is swallowed, the larva is released by digestion, attaches itself to the mucosa, and grows into an adult. Children are infected accidentally by swallowing infected fleas when handling dogs.

Clinical picture and treatment

Infection usually occurs in young children and is often asymptomatic. Diarrhoea and allergic reactions are sometimes caused. Niclosamide as used for *T. saginata* is effective.

Coenurus

In addition, there are two species of the taeniid worm *Multiceps* whose intermediate stages produce rare and accidental infections in man. These intermediate stages are characterized by the presence of numerous scoleces in a single bladder, and are referred to as 'coenuri'.

Coenurus cerebralis is only rarely found as a parasite of man. The adult tapeworm, *Multiceps multiceps*, occurs only in carnivores, mainly in dogs. The larval stage usually occurs in herbivorous animals, mainly sheep and goats, but it is occasionally recorded in man. The hexacanth embryo invades nervous tissue, frequently the brain, and instead of producing a single scolex as in a cysticercus it produces a number of heads invaginated into a common bladder, which may be 5–6 cm in diameter (Fig. 5.3).

Coenurus serialis is the larval stage of *Multiceps serialis*, which occurs as an adult in the small intestine of dogs. The larval stage develops in the intermuscular connective tissue of rabbits and hares, and occasionally produces cysts the size of a hen's egg in the human host. *C. serialis* can be distinguished from *C. cerebralis* by its location in the muscles, and by the fact that the numerous scoleces in the cyst are arranged in lines radiating from a centre (Fig. 5.3). An additional difference is that *C. serialis* may form daughter cysts inside or outside the main cyst, and these may produce scoleces. In this respect the coenurus resembles the hydatid cyst.

Clinical picture and treatment

Coenurosis is a rare disease in man causing invasion of cerebral, eye or subcutaneous tissues. The clinical picture is similar to that of cysticercosis. Prognosis when a cyst occurs in the brain is grave — surgery is usually not possible. In sheep, cerebral coenurosis is more common, causing the 'staggers'.

Family Hymenolepididae

This family of the Cyclophyllidea is also of medical importance, and contains one species of tapeworm which, although not obviously pathogenic, occurs sufficiently commonly in man to render its recognition important. The members of the family are easily recognized. The segments are always broader than they are long; instead of numerous testes (as occur in the Taeniidae) there are never more than four, and usually only three; and the genital pores are unilateral.

Hymenolepis nana

This species is sometimes called the 'dwarf tapeworm' because it is the smallest adult tapeworm occurring in man. The strobila generally does not exceed 2–3 cm in length, and is made up of more than 100 segments, each measuring about 500–800 μm broad and 250 μm long (Fig. 5.2). The unilateral genital pores open in the anterior corner of each proglottis. The head is small and globular, and is armed with a single row of about 28 hooks, each measuring about 16 μm, mounted on a retractile rostellum (Fig. 5.1).

The adult worm tends to occur more frequently in children than in adults. Its distribution is more or less world-wide, but it is particularly common in the Mediterranean area. It occurs in man and in domestic rodents, rats and mice. The human strain appears to be different biologically from the rodent strain; the human strain usually passes directly from man to man, although man can also (with difficulty) be infected with the rodent strain. In man no intermediate host is required, so that, as in infections with *T. solium*, the patient can directly infect his neighbours and also reinfect himself.

Hymenolepis nana is an exception to the general rule that helminths do not multiply inside the definitive host. When the egg is swallowed by man the hexacanth embryo escapes in the small intestine, burrows into the mucosa of a villus, and develops into a cysticercoid. The cysticercoid differs from a cysticercus in that liquefaction of the oncosphere is slight, and the resultant fluid is soon absorbed so that in the infective stage there is no bladder. When the armed head is completely formed it evaginates, and the cysticercoid then ruptures through the villus back into the lumen of the gut, and there attaches itself to the gut wall and buds off new segments.

The development in rats and mice is similar, but in rodent strains the cysticercoid usually develops in an intermediate arthropod host, such as a flea or beetle larva.

Clinical picture and treatment

This common infection is usually found in children and is normally asymptomatic. Very heavy infections cause diarrhoea and abdominal pain. General manifestations such as headache, irritability and allergic symptoms have also been ascribed to this worm.

Niclosamide is used in treatment, and because of the nature of the life-cycle it should be given for a week, 2 g on day 1 and then 1 g daily for six days; for children, the dosages should be as described for infections with *T. saginata* (see p. 89).

Hymenolepis diminuta

Another species of *Hymenolepis, H. diminuta*, is a very common parasite of rats and mice, but very rarely occurs in man. The adult has an unarmed head, measures 10–60 mm in length (larger than *H. nana*), and has anything up to 1000 segments. The larval stages are usually found in the haemocoele of insects, principally fleas and cockroaches.

Order Pseudophyllidea

Parasites belonging to this Order are characterized by having a scolex that possesses sucking grooves or 'bothria' instead of circular suckers, and by not having any hooks. The segments are broader than they are long, the genital pore is situated on the flat surface of the segment, and the uterus opens to the exterior by a small pore which is also on the flat surface of the segment. There is only one species of medical importance in the Order, namely *Diphyllobothrium latum*.

Diphyllobothrium latum

The adult tapeworm occurs in the small intestine of man and fish-eating animals such as cats, dogs and bears. It has a world-wide distribution, occurring in the vicinity of most of the great lakes of the world. It grows to a great length, usually 3–4 metres but sometimes up to 10 metres, and its maximum breadth is about 2 cm. There may be over 3000 segments. The head is almond-shaped, with two sucking grooves, and there is a very long neck (Fig. 5.1). The uterus opens to the exterior by means of the uterine pore, and the eggs are continually being passed out into the lumen of the small intestine from the segments — the gravid segments are retained longer than those of the Taeniidae. As a result, there are usually enormous numbers of eggs in the faeces, and the infection can easily be recognized by microscopic examination of the faeces. The eggs are fertilized when passed, but unlike those of the Taeniidae and Hymenolepididae are undeveloped and noninfective. When passed the eggs are tightly packed with globular cells, one of which develops at the expense of the others into a true ovum — but this development only takes place in water after the egg is passed. Full development requires about 2 weeks for its completion. The ovum, during this period, develops into a hexacanth embryo, enclosed in an embryophore just as in the other tapeworms; but in *D. latum* the appearance and the arrangement of the various layers of the egg are quite different. In the genera *Taenia* and *Echinococcus* the ova are indistinguishable and possess a very thin outer egg shell and a very delicate vitelline membrane, both of which usually vanish early in the life-cycle to leave only the thick striated embryophore enclosing the hexacanth embryo (see Fig. 9.2). In *Hymenolepis* there is a moderately developed true egg shell enclosing a semisolid transparent yolk layer surrounding an embryophore that is unstriated and relatively thin (see Fig. 9.2). In *Diphyllobothrium latum* the thin egg shell has been replaced by a thick, strong, operculated shell containing a delicate vitelline membrane, and the embryophore has become ciliated. But although the layers of protective covering have been altered in each of these genera and adapted to the needs of the enclosed hexacanth embryo, the embryo itself is essentially the same in each instance.

About 2 weeks after being passed in the faeces the larva of *D. latum* is completely formed. It then pushes off the cap at the end of the egg, ruptures the delicate vitelline membrane, and enters the water. It swims, or rather is carried about by the ciliated embryophore. The combined embryo and embryophore is called a 'coracidium'. Sometimes the embryo bursts out of its ciliated covering and sinks to the bottom of the water, where it is capable of creeping about — but whether or not it remains inside the embryophore, it dies within about 24 hours unless it is swallowed by the correct intermediate host.

The correct intermediate host is a freshwater crustacean belonging to the genus *Cyclops* or *Diaptomus*. If the coracidium is ingested by one of these water fleas the ciliated embryophore is lost and the hexacanth embryo burrows through the gut wall into the body cavity. Once there, it develops within 2–3 weeks into the 'procercoid', which is an early stage of development of a cysticercoid with an elongated shape and in which the scolex is not yet developed.

The larva does not develop further until the crustacean is eaten by a freshwater fish — pike and perch seem the most suitable. Inside the fish the crustacean and the terminal part of the procercoid are digested, but the main part of the procercoid migrates into the body cavity of the fish and becomes transformed into a 'plerocercoid'. The fully developed plerocercoid has what is obviously a tapeworm head with sucking grooves, and a longish unsegmented tail (Fig. 5.3). Mature plerocercoids may be anything from 6 mm to 2 cm in length, and are distributed throughout the muscles of the fish. The plerocercoid is the infective stage, and the final host (including man) becomes infected by eating the plerocercoid in raw or undercooked fish. The adult cestode becomes mature in 2–4 weeks after the infective meal, and has a potential life of about 5 years.

Pathogenesis and clinical picture

These large tapeworms inhabit the jejunum or ileum and generally cause no symptoms. Sometimes the infestation causes abdominal discomfort, vomiting and weight loss. Rarely intestinal obstruction occurs as a result of multiple infection. *D. latum* splits the vitamin B_{12}-intrinsic factor compound in the gut and can utilize 80–100 per cent of the host's ingested vitamin B_{12} if it is attached high in the jejunum. There is also interference with folate absorption. In less than 2 per cent of those infected, Addisonian pernicious anaemia and, less commonly, subacute combined degeneration result. Overt B_{12} deficiency is much more common in Finland than elsewhere.

Diagnosis and treatment

Segments are not usually passed in the stools, but ova are found in the stools. Haematological investigations are needed to assess anaemia and vitamin B_{12} status.

Niclosamide is used as for *T. saginata*. Intramuscular cyanocobalamin is given if there is vitamin B_{12} deficiency.

Sparganum

Zoologically, the term sparganum is synonymous with plerocercoid, but in medical helminthology it is particularly applied to a diphyllobothrioid plerocercoid of unknown origin found in man. These infections are given the medical name of sparganosis. Infections with sparganum are accidental, man not being the normal second intermediate host for the tapeworm concerned — and frequently the sparganum cannot in our present state of knowledge be related to its adult tapeworm, nor is its full life-history known.

Probably the best known sparganum is that which was first named *Sparganum mansoni*. (*Sparganum*, of course, is not a generic name in the normal sense.) *Sp. mansoni* is widely distributed in the Far East, and cases have been reported from the USA. It has now been identified as the larval stage of *Spirometra mansoni*, which occurs as an adult in the small intestine of dogs and cats. The normal life-history is that the eggs are passed in the faeces of the host and the procercoid develops in the water flea *Cyclops*. The plerocercoid normally develops in frogs, snakes, birds or mammals which ingest infected *Cyclops*, and the adult develops when any of these are eaten by dogs or cats. Only the plerocercoid stage develops in man (as sparganum). Man is presumably infected by accidentally swallowing an infected *Cyclops*, but it has been suggested that in primitive communities infection can follow eating raw infected snake meat, or applying a plerocercoid-infected host as a poultice to an open lesion.

Another sparganum, *Sp. proliferum*, is found mainly in Japan, but occurs rarely and sporadically elsewhere. The life-history of the parasite is unknown, but man probably acquires the infection from eating raw fish. The sparganum is found in large numbers in the subcutaneous tissues, muscles and internal organs — in swellings and cysts like *Sp. mansoni*. The young plerocercoid or sparganum measures about 3 mm in length by 300 µm in breadth. The fully grown larva measures about 12 × 2.5 mm. The anterior end is narrower than the posterior, and frequently the larva proliferates to form supernumerary buds which may become detached, each to form a separate cyst.

Clinical picture

Sparganosis presents as a painful subcutaneous swelling. The lump may spontaneously disappear, only to recur at some other site; i.e. the plerocercoid has migrated. The orbital tissues, and subcutaneous tissues on the torso, limbs and scrotum, are often involved. More seriously, lesions rarely appear in the nervous system, abdomen and pleura. The subcutaneous lesions are erythematous, itchy and painful, and may suppurate.

The diagnosis is often made when the plerocercoid larva is identified in tissues removed at operation. No drug is effective and surgical removal is the only treatment.

Laboratory identification of cestodes

Human infections with adult tapeworms are identified by the finding of either gravid segments or eggs (or occasionally both) in the faeces. Immature segments are frequently unidentifiable to species — but these do not normally occur in faeces. Scoleces, or large pieces of tapeworms, are found only after treatment and purges. In infections with *Taenia* spp. (and the rare *Dipylidium*) eggs are found in the faeces only when the gravid segment disintegrates before it is passed; this occurs in about one quarter of cases. In most cases the gravid segments are unruptured when passed in the faeces, and consequently individual eggs are not found. In infections with *Diphyllobothrium* (and with *Hymenolepis* spp.) eggs are normally liberated in the intestine and passed with the faeces.

Identification of gravid segments (Fig. 5.2)

The tapeworms that occur commonly in man can readily be identified from a single gravid segment, if one is found. Freshly passed segments are very active and muscular, and constantly changing in shape, so that individual segments may show considerable differences in form from the average description given here.

Taenia solium segments

The gravid segment measures about 1.5 cm long and about 0.8 cm wide. The genital pore is single, on the lateral margin of the segment. The segment can be identified by the shape of the gravid uterus, which can usually be seen if the segment is pressed between two glass plates and held up to the light. The uterus cannot be seen if all the contained eggs have escaped, but this difficulty can be overcome by injecting waterproof drawing ink (Indian ink or Chinese ink) into the empty uterus. Alternatively, the segment can be fixed and cleared, or it can be stained. The gravid uterus of *T. solium* consists of a median stem with 4–12 lateral compound branches on each side. When counting the branches, only the main stems should be counted and the confused branching at the anterior and posterior ends of the median stem should be ignored.

Taenia saginata segments

The gravid segment measures about 2 cm long and about 0.5 cm wide, and is generally similar in form to that of *T. solium*. The gravid uterus shows 15–30 lateral compound branches on each side, which distinguishes the segment from that of *T. solium*.

Hymenolepis nana segments

The gravid segment measures about 0.3 mm long and about 1 mm wide. The genital pore is single, on the lateral margin of the segment. Segments rarely appear in the faeces, but if they do they are usually associated as small lengths of strobila rather than occurring singly. *Hymenolepis* segments can be recognized by their small size.

Hymenolepis diminuta segments

The gravid segment measures about 0.7 mm long and about 2.5 mm wide, and is generally similar in form to that of *H. nana*. As in infections with *H. nana*, segments rarely appear in the faeces, and if they do they are usually attached to each other as small lengths of worm.

Dipylidium caninum segments

The gravid segment measures about 5 mm long and about 2.5 mm wide, and is characterized by being rather barrel-shaped and by having a genital pore on each margin. The segment appears reticulated because the uterus is divided into numerous uterine 'pockets'.

Diphyllobothrium latum segments

The gravid segment measures about 0.4 cm long and about 1.5 cm wide. The genital pore is on the flat surface of the segment. The gravid uterus is creamy-yellow and appears as a darker rosette-shaped body in the centre of the ivory-coloured segment.

Identification of eggs

The eggs of tapeworm parasites of man can also be readily identified, except that the eggs of the two species of *Taenia* are morphologically indistinguishable.

Taenia solium and *T. saginata* eggs (see Fig.9.2)

Taenia eggs are not commonly found in faeces, gravid segments being more common. The egg shell is very delicate, and contains the embryo and yolk cells. The egg shell and yolk cells are usually lost when the egg leaves the proglottis; and the 'egg', when seen in the faeces, is brown, spherical or ovoid, and about 35 μm in diameter. It consists of a thick striated embryophore enclosing the 'hexacanth embryo'. The six hooks of the embryo can easily be seen in the living eggs, but they are usually obscured in preserved eggs.

Hymenolepis nana eggs (see Fig. 9.2)

The eggs are colourless and transparent, and usually ovoid in shape. The vary in length from 30 μm to 50 μm, and contain a hexacanth embryo about 18 μm in diameter covered by a thin embryophore. At each end of the embryophore is a small knob or thickening, and from each of these arises a group of 4–8 long, thin 'polar filaments'. The eggs are normally liberated in the intestine and passed with the faeces.

Hymenolepis diminuta eggs

The eggs are yellow or golden and only slightly ovoid, and the egg shell may show fine striations. They vary in size from 60 μm to 85 μm, and contain a hexacanth embryo about 25 μm in diameter. At each end of the embryophore is a polar knob, but there are no polar filaments.

Dipylidium caninum eggs

The eggs are similar in size and structure to those of *Taenia solium* and *T. saginata*, except that they are usually spherical and light brick-red in colour. Normally gravid proglottids are passed in the faeces, but if the gravid proglottis ruptures then the eggs are found in small groups of 5–30 eggs (usually about 12) enclosed in a common membrane. Each of these packets of eggs represents a pocket of the gravid uterus.

Diphyllobothrium latum eggs (Fig. 9.2)

The eggs are ovoid, with a fairly thick wall and a small lid or 'operculum' at one end. They are yellowish-brown, about 70 μm long and 45 μm wide. When passed in the faeces the egg contains a fertilized undeveloped ovum surrounded by yolk cells. The operculum (which is characteristic of trematode eggs rather then cestode eggs) is difficult to see in freshly passed eggs, but becomes more conspicuous as the larva develops and becomes ready for hatching.

Identification of larval cestodes

In addition to the tapeworms that infect man in their adult stages, there are some which may infect man in their larval stages. Such infections are accidental, man taking the place of the normal intermediate host, and the larval stages cannot complete the life-cycle and grow into adults. Identification of these infections is normally outside the range of usual laboratory work, but excised cestode larvae are usually recognizable.

Cysticerci (Fig. 5.3)

A cysticercus is the 'bladder-worm' stage of a taeniid tapeworm which contains a single scolex; and the only one which normally infects man is *Cysticercus cellulosae*, the larval stage of *Taenia solium*. A few cases of human infection with *C. bovis*, the larval stage of *T. saginata*, have been recorded. The normal host of *C. cellulosae* is the pig, and man becomes infected by swallowing the egg of *T. solium*, often by autoinfection. Cysticerci may occur in practically every organ and tissue of the body. An excised larva can be identified by its small size (up to 1 cm in diameter) and its single invaginated scolex, which is armed with four suckers and a ring of typical taeniid hooks like those of the adult. The scolex of *C. bovis*, like that of the parent *T. saginata*, bears no hooks.

Coenuri (Fig. 5.3)

The coenurus is a cestode bladder stage in which several scoleces are formed as invaginations of a single cyst; and the main ones that have been reported in man are *Coenurus cerebralis* (the larval stage of *Multiceps multiceps*) and *C. serialis* (the larval stage of *M. serialis*). The adult *Multiceps* is a parasite of canines, and the normal hosts of the coenuri are herbivores. Man is infected accidentally, usually by ingesting eggs passed by domestic dogs. A coenurus is about 5 cm in diameter, and can be identified by the presence of numerous scoleces, each armed with suckers and hooks like those of the adult. The scoleces of *C. cerebralis* are scattered irregularly over the bladder, while those of *C. serialis* are arranged in lines radiating from a centre.

Hydatid cysts

A hydatid cyst is a cestode bladder stage in which the bladder is invaginated into numerous 'brood capsules', each of which is further invaginated to form scoleces. There are two species of tapeworms, *Echinococcus granulosus* and *E. multilocularis*, that occur in man in the larval stage as hydatid cysts. The adult worms are parasites of carnivores, and the larval stages normally occur in herbivores. Man is accidentally infected by ingesting eggs, usually those passed by domestic dogs, and hydatid cysts may develop in various organs and tissues, especially the liver and lungs. They are normally 5–10 cm in diameter, but in man may grow as large as 50 cm. Hydatid cysts may be fertile (with scoleces) or sterile (without scoleces). Fertile cysts contain large numbers of free brood capsules and scoleces, which are collectively referred to as 'hydatid sand'. This is identifiable by the presence of brood capsules, scoleces and taeniid hooks, and its presence in the aspirated fluid of a cyst proves the cyst to be that of *Echinococcus*.

Spargana (Fig. 5.3)

A sparganum is the plerocercoid stage of a diphyllobothrioid tapeworm that develops accidentally in man. The normal hosts of plerocercoids are lower vertebrates. There is some doubt as to how man becomes infected, and several possible methods have been suggested. A sparganum is a small, white, ribbon-shaped larva, which may be up to a few centimetres in length, and may be found in the subcutaneous tissue or in the deeper organs of the body. After excision they can be recognized by their typical plerocercoid structure.

General principles of tapeworm control

With one notable exception, tapeworm infections in man can be divided into adult infections, caused by the ingestion of the larval stage of the worm in the muscle or body cavity of an intermediate host, and larval infections, caused by the ingestion of the egg in contaminated food or drink. An exception is *Hymenolepis nana*, in which ingestion of the egg gives rise to a larval stage that further develops to the adult stage, and so results in an adult infection.

Ingestion of the larval stage

The important worms transmitted in this way are the three large tapeworms, *Taenia solium, T. saginata* and *Diphyllobothrium latum*, transmitted respectively by infected muscle of pigs, cattle and fish. These animals become infected by ingesting eggs passed in human faeces or (for *Diphyllobothrium* but not *Taenia*) in the faeces of man or of 'reservoir' hosts. Obviously *Taenia* infections would be less common if cattle and pigs were prevented from feeding or grazing on ground contaminated by human faeces, but such prevention has proved difficult even in 'developed' countries. It is not possible to prevent eggs of *Diphyllobothrium* from contaminating bodies of fresh water, especially as eggs often come from sources other than human. Infections in pigs, cattle and fish are thus extremely difficult to prevent.

All beef and pork destined for human consumption should be examined for cysticerci, and this is done in countries where meat inspection is routine. Heavily infected carcasses are condemned as unfit for human consumption, but lightly infected carcasses may be frozen (say at −21°C for 21 days) to kill the cysticerci and then released for food. However, the cysticerci are small and there are practical limits to how far a carcass can be mutilated, so some very light infections will be missed by the meat inspectors. Fish are not normally inspected. Prevention of infection thus depends mainly on the proper cooking of meat and fish. Cysticerci and plerocercoids are killed at about 56°C, but it must be remembered that a cooking temperature much higher than this is required to kill tapeworm larvae in the centre of a thick piece of muscle.

Some infections with adult tapeworms follow ingestion of the larval stage in an arthropod. Ingestion of fleas may produce infection with *Dipylidium caninum* or *Hymenolepis diminuta*, which are recorded infrequently in man, and several rare parasites are transmitted in fleas, cockroaches and mites. Infection with any of the arthropod-borne tapeworms is accidental, and usually occurs in childhood; prevention of infection depends on personal hygiene.

Ingestion of the egg

The ingestion by man of certain tapeworm eggs may lead to infection with the larval stages, with man accidentally taking the place of the normal intermediate host of the tapeworm. Examples of this are cysticercosis, hydatid disease, coenuriasis and sparganosis, caused respectively by the ingestion of eggs of *Taenia solium, Echinococcus* spp., *Multiceps* spp. and some diphyllobothrioid worms.

Ingestion of the eggs of *Hymenolepis nana* leads first to infection with the larval stages, and then to infection with the adult worm when the larval stages develop. *H. nana* is exceptional in that the one person acts both as intermediate host and final host.

Prevention of Infection

This depends mainly on good standards of personal hygiene, sanitation and health education. Most infections probably arise from the ingestion of contaminated food (particularly vegetables) or water, although eggs of *T. solium* can be carried directly on soiled fingers to produce auto-infection, and perhaps infection of other members of the household. In a similar manner, where dogs are household pets or are otherwise closely associated with man, hydatid infections (especially of children) may follow the ingestion of eggs which contaminate the fingers of individuals playing with or otherwise handling the dog.

Further reading

von Bonsdorff B. Diphyllobothriasis in man, London: Academic Press, 1977.
Jones TC. Cestodes. *Clin Gastroenterol* 1978 **7**: 105–28.
Lawson JR, Gemmell MA. Hydatidosis and cysticercosis: the dynamics of transmission. *Adv Parasitol* 1983, **22**: 261–308.
Muller R. Worms and disease. London: Heinemann, 1975.
Pawlowski Z. Cestode infections. In: Warren KS and Mahmoud AAf (eds) *Tropical and geographical medicine*. New York: McGraw-Hill, 1984; 471–86.
Pawlowski Z, Schultz MG. Taeniasis and cysticercosis (*Taenia saginata*). *Adv. Parasitol* 1972; **10**: 269–308.

6
Flukes

The class Trematoda, commonly called trematodes or flukes, can be distinguished from the class Cestoda, commonly called cestodes or tapeworms, by the following points. A cestode possesses a distinct head, which bears sucking organs, and consists of a chain of segments; it has no intestine, and is a hermaphrodite. A trematode possesses no distinct head; the body is unsegmented, and usually has two suckers; there is an intestine. Most trematodes are hermaphrodites, but in some the sexes are separate.

The trematodes parasitizing man vary in size, according to the species, from the tiny — just visible — *Heterophyes* to the relatively large *Fasciolopsis*, which may be up to 7 cm in length. Individuals of the same species also vary in size, according to their maturity and food supply. The majority of the Trematoda are flattened, and oval or leaf-like in outline, as are *Fasciola* and *Clonorchis*; but some are thread-like, as is *Schistosoma*, or fleshy, like *Heterophyes* and *Paragonimus*.

It may be said, in the most general terms, that the species which parasitize man have their adult stage in the human host, while the next stage develops in various species of molluscs, from which the larvae later emerge and either invade man directly or else pass through another intermediate encysted stage, either in crustacea, in fish or on vegetation. This form of development is referred to as 'digenetic', as distinct from 'monogenetic' which implies development without an intermediate host. All the trematodes parasitizing man have a digenetic life-cycle.

Class Trematoda

The Trematoda show certain well-marked differences in their morphology and life-cycle, and in consequence they can be divided into various superfamilies. Four of these superfamilies include parasites of man, and these are the Echinostomatoidea, the Opisthorchioidea, the Plagiorchioidea and the Schistosomatoidea. However, the general morphology and histology, and the basic life-cycle, of members of all these superfamilies have much in common, so it is possible to consider the general structure (Fig. 6.1) and development of the trematodes as a whole.

The adult trematode usually possesses two suckers, one oral surrounding the mouth and one ventral lying on the median line. The body is covered with an integument on which spines are sometimes present; if present the spines are most marked on the anterior half of the body. Underlying the integument is a layer of muscle fibres, by means of which the animal can alter its shape, move about, and squeeze its way into and through narrow apertures.

The mouth opens into the pharynx, behind which is the oesophagus which branches into two blind-ending caeca. The excretory system, like the gut, is bilaterally symmetrical. It consists of a series of flame cells, which drive waste fluids into collecting tubules, which connect with capillaries, which in their turn drain into two main collecting channels which open into a posteriorly placed bladder.

In all superfamilies of the Trematoda, with the exception of the Schistosomatoidea, the male and female sex organs occur in the same individual. In these hermaphrodite trematodes the sex organs are arranged on the same general principle as are those of the tapeworms. The male sexual organs usually consist of two testes, from each of which a vas efferens leads to a single vas deferens. This enters the cirrus sac and becomes enlarged and convoluted to form a seminal vesicle. The cirrus is protrusible through the genital pore, which is situated above and to one side of the ventral sucker.

The female genital organs consist of a single ovary, with an oviduct leading to a tubular structure, the ootype, which is the chamber where the eggs are fertilized and where all the components of the egg are collected. From the ootype leads a tube serving the double purpose of a vagina (for receiving the spermatozoa) and a uterus (in which the fertilized eggs are stored), which is usually referred to by the latter name. This uterus passes forward and opens at the genital pore beside the cirrus, from which it receives the sperms. There are other structures surrounding the ootype. On the dorsal side there is usually a flask-shaped structure where the spermatozoa are stored, and which is called the seminal receptacle. Opening into the seminal receptacle is another structure known as Laurer's canal, the function of which is not known (but it opens on the dorsal surface of the body and probably functions as an aid to cross-fertilization). Surrounding the ootype is a cluster of glands forming Mehlis' organ, which is possibly associated with the formation of the egg shell. The yolk glands, or vitellaria, lie along the margins of the body, and the ducts from the glands open into the ootype.

The adult trematodes parasitizing man occur in the body in a variety of sites. If they occur in the lumen of the gut, in the veins surrounding the gut, or in the bile ducts, the eggs are passed in the faeces. If they are in the veins surrounding the bladder, the eggs ulcerate through the walls and are passed in the urine. Some trematodes occur in the lungs, in which case the eggs reach the outside world in the sputum, or if swallowed, in the faeces.

Superfamily Echinostomatoidea

The members of this superfamily are large flattened flukes, living in the intestine and biliary ducts of man and various animals, including domestic animals. They are all hermaphrodites. The reproductive organs are generally as described above, and the testes are large and branched. The eggs are large, operculated, and contain an undeveloped ovum when passed.

Three genera of the superfamily are described as parasitizing man. Two of these, *Fasciola* and *Echinostoma*, are uncommon human parasites; but the third, *Fasciolopsis*, is a common and widely distributed pathogenic parasite of man.

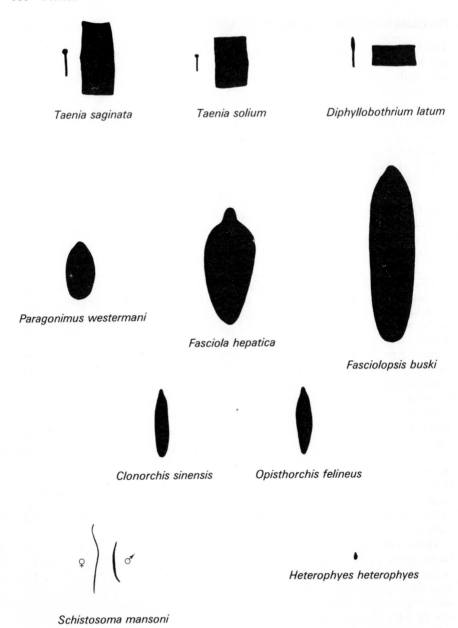

Taenia saginata   *Taenia solium*   *Diphyllobothrium latum*

Paragonimus westermani

Fasciola hepatica

Fasciolopsis buski

Clonorchis sinensis   *Opisthorchis felineus*

Heterophyes heterophyes

♀   ♂

Schistosoma mansoni

Fig. 6.1   Actual sizes of common Platyhelminth parasites of Man. For each Cestode parasite, the head and one gravid segment are shown: for each Trematode parasite, the complete worm is shown.

Fasciolopsis buski (Fig. 6.1)

This fluke is essentially confined to the Far East. It is common in Japan, China and Korea, and its range extends southwards to India, Borneo and Malaysia. The adult forms occur in man and in pigs; other animals can become infected but do not act as reservoirs. In their natural hosts, man and the pig, the adults can be found attached by their ventral suckers to the mucosa of the small intestine, particularly in the duodenum.

Fasciolopsis buski is the largest trematode commonly parasitizing man. It is a thick fleshy oval fluke, about 2–7 cm in length and 1–2 cm in breadth (Fig. 6.1). Morphologically it closely resembles *Fasciola hepatica*, the common liver fluke of sheep, which has a world-wide distribution. *Fasciolopsis* has a body wall armed with spines, but these are easily lost and are often absent from preserved specimens. The arrangement of the internal organs is basically similar to that described above for the class as a whole.

The life-cycle is typical of digenetic trematodes. The egg, when passed in the faeces, measures about 140×80 μm, is oval, and has a clear thick shell with a small operculum at one end. The egg contains a fertilized but unsegmented ovum, surrounded by yolk cells (see Fig. 9.2). Further development takes place in water, and after about a month at optimum temperature a ciliated larva or miracidium is formed. This larva then pushes off the operculum and swims free in the water. It has a life span of about two days in optimum conditions. If during this time it encounters a suitable molluscan host (a snail of the genus *Hippeutis* or *Segmentina*), the miracidium penetrates through the body wall of the snail. The miracidium then migrates in the haemocoele, and, if it reaches the digestive gland, develops into the next larval stage, the sporocyst. The sporocyst is a simply-organized sacculate body, and the cells lining the cavity proliferate to produce small masses of cells known as germ balls. Each germ ball develops into another type of larva, the redia. The sporocyst now ruptures and liberates the rediae, inside each of which further germ balls are produced. These may develop into further generations of rediae (called daughter rediae), the number of generations depending on various factors such as the food supply. Finally the rediae (or daughter rediae) produce within themselves the final (infective) larval stage, the cercariae. These escape from the rediae, burrow through the tissue of the snail, and emerge into the water. The development in the snail takes 4–8 weeks.

The cercaria consists of an anterior oval portion on which the suckers of the future adult can be distinguished, and a tail-like structure by means of which it swims (Fig. 6.2). The cercariae can survive for about 24 hours, and within this time they encyst on various water plants. The encysted stages are known as metacercariae, and are found on certain species of water plants that are eaten raw by both pigs and man, such as the fruit of the water chestnut, *Eliocharis tuberosa*, and the root and tuber of the water caltrop, *Trapa natans* or *T. bicornis*. Man and pigs become infected when they ingest the metacercariae.

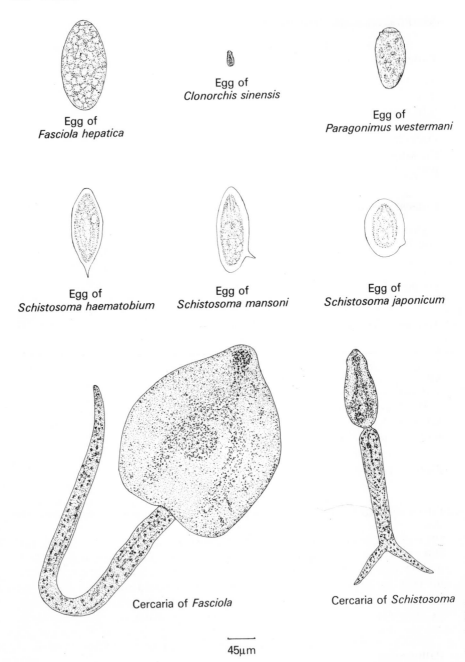

Egg of
Fasciola hepatica

Egg of
Clonorchis sinensis

Egg of
Paragonimus westermani

Egg of
Schistosoma haematobium

Egg of
Schistosoma mansoni

Egg of
Schistosoma japonicum

Cercaria of *Fasciola*

Cercaria of *Schistosoma*

45μm

Fig. 6.2 Immature stages of Trematodes.

Medical aspects of *F. buski* infections

Pathogenesis

This large fluke is attached to the mucosa of the small intestine and may cause ulceration, abscess formation and haemorrhage at the site of attachment. Most infections are light, with 10–20 worm pairs, but heavier infections with anything from 100 to over 1000 worm pairs in children cause serious and even fatal illness. Oedema of the face and ascites occur, possibly due to some toxic metabolite of the worm, but hypoalbuminaemia due to protein-losing enteropathy may play a part.

Clinical picture

Light infections are usually asymptomatic; heavier infections in poorly nourished children are associated with abdominal pain (sometimes eased by food), intermittent diarrhoea and a clinical picture resembling protein–calorie malnutrition with oedema, ascites and wasting. Intestinal obstruction due to paralytic ileus is an occasional complication.

Treatment and prevention

Hexylresorcinol in doses of 1 g for subjects over the age of 7 years, and 400 mg for younger children, has been effective, as has tetrachlorethylene 0.12 ml/kg up to a maximum of 5 ml. Praziquantel in a dose of 15 mg/kg body weight given at bedtime has been found effective in Thailand.

Water plants such as the water caltrop should be cooked before being eaten (or at least adequately peeled), and not taken from ponds contaminated with human or pig faeces.

Fasciola hepatica

This trematode is widespread in sheep-raising areas. The adults live in the bile ducts, and are common in sheep, goats and cattle, less common in horses and pigs, and uncommon in man. The adult worm differs from *Fasciolopsis* in that the caeca of the alimentary canal are branched, and the 'shoulders' at the anterior end are more definite (Fig. 6.1). The intermediate snail host is *Lymnaea*, and the metacercariae are encysted on blades of grass on the wet pastures. The infection causes 'liver rot' in sheep, and may cause liver damage in man.

Medical aspects of *F. hepatica* infection (fascioliasis)

Pathogenesis

F. hepatica reaches the bile ducts by penetrating the liver surface after traversing the small intestinal wall and peritoneal cavity. The larvae may be destroyed in the liver substance, causing an inflammatory mass. The adult worm lives in large bile ducts, causing inflammation, some periportal fibrosis and sometimes significant haemorrhage in the ducts (haemobilia). Serious pathology is rare, and only occurs in heavy infections. Larval worms have occasionally migrated to subcutaneous tissues, brain and lungs.

Clinical picture and diagnosis

In the early stages there is right hypochondrium pain, tender hepatomegaly, fever, urticaria and eosinophilia. Generally these symptoms gradually subside over the course of a few months. In severe chronic cases there may be recurrent jaundice, fever, vomiting and anaemia due to haemobilia. Cirrhosis and portal hypertension probably do not occur. Subcutaneous fascioliasis presents as migrating painful subcutaneous nodules.

Fascioliasis must be differentiated from other causes of upper abdominal pain, tender hepatomegaly and jaundice. These causes include virus hepatitis, amoebic liver abscess, cholecystitis and primary biliary cirrhosis. The combination of hepatomegaly, eosinophilia and a raised serum alkaline phosphatase is suggestive of liver fluke infection.

Treatment

Bithionol 100 mg/kg is given orally on alternate days for 2–3 weeks. Emetine hydrochloride in doses of 30 mg IM daily for 15 days has also been used. Praziquantel is not very effective in this infection.

'Halzoun'

This is an acute inflammation of the nasopharynx following attachment of certain parasites to the pharynx after eating raw liver. There is pain in the throat, coughing, sneezing, nasal discharge and dysphagia. Spontaneous recovery ensues in 7–10 days, but rare cases of fatal asphyxiation have been recorded. *Fasciola* was thought to be a common cause of halzoun, but it is now considered to be usually due to nymphs of the pentastomid worm *Linguatula serrata* or to leeches such as *Limnatis nilotica*.

Superfamily Opisthorchioidea

Members of this superfamily are flattened transparent medium-sized flukes, the adults of which live in the biliary ducts. They are all hermaphrodites whose eggs, when seen in the faeces, are small and operculated and contain a developed miracidium. The first larval stages occur in freshwater snails, the final larval stage is encysted in freshwater fishes, and the adults develop in mammals that have ingested the larvae when eating the fish.

Only one species in this superfamily commonly occurs in man, *Clonorchis sinensis*. Another species, *Opisthorchis felineus*, which is normally parasitic in cats, is a not-uncommon parasite of man in Siberia and parts of India and Europe, and *O. viverrini* is an important parasite in man in Thailand.

Clonorchis sinensis

This fluke, which is also known as *Opisthorchis sinensis*, is essentially confined to the Far East, and is common in certain parts of Japan, China, Korea and Indo-China. The adult forms occur in these countries not only in man but also in domestic animals, particularly cats and dogs, which form an important animal reservoir. The flukes usually inhabit the bile passages in the liver, but are sometimes found in the pancreatic duct.

The adult worm varies greatly in size, but is usually 1–2 cm in length and 0.15–0.5 cm in breadth (Fig. 6.1). It is a rather transparent, flattened worm, usually spoon-shaped and usually yellow-brown owing to bile staining. Its structure is fairly typical, except that the branched testes are arranged one in front of the other; this tandem arrangement is characteristic of the species. The eggs, when seen in the faeces, are yellowish-brown flask-shaped structures, about 30 μm long and 15 μm broad (Fig. 9.2). Each contains a ciliated miracidium, but this larva is not liberated until the egg is ingested by a freshwater snail belonging to one of several genera including *Bulimus, Parafossarulus* and *Melanoides*. The egg hatches in the oesophagus of the snail and releases the miracidium, which penetrates the gut wall and passes into the haemocoele. Development proceeds in the normal way through sporocysts, rediae and cercariae, and the cercariae emerge from the snail. The cercaria leads a free existence in the water, but dies in about 24 hours unless it comes into contact with its next intermediate host, which is a fish. If it reaches a fish belonging to the correct species — probably many families can be parasitized — it burrows beneath the scales and discards its tail. It may encyst beneath the scales or in the skin or muscle of the fish.

If man eats raw or improperly cooked or pickled fish containing the metacercaria of *C. sinensis*, the cyst wall is dissolved in the duodenum and the miniature fluke works its way through the intestinal opening into the common bile duct, where it grows to maturity. The mature worm begins to lay eggs about 4 weeks after ingestion. The total life-cycle probably occupies about 4 or 5 months.

Medical aspects of *C. sinesis* infection (clonorchiasis)

Pathogenesis

Larvae ascend the common bile duct from the small intestine, reach medium-sized bile ducts, and there mature into adults. In the bile ducts the long-lived flukes (up to 24 years) act as irritants, provoking goblet-cell hyperplasia, excess mucous secretion and metaplasia of the bile duct epithelium which may become neoplastic. Inflammation round the ducts, fibrosis and dead worms cause biliary obstruction, duct dilatation and diverticula formation. Consequences of these changes are bacterial cholangitis and intrahepatic biliary stone formation. Fibriotic changes may occlude portal venous radicles. In heavily infected cases a type of secondary biliary cirrhosis and portal hypertension may develop, as may cholangiocarcinoma. Flukes can invade pancreatic ducts and cause pancreatitis.

Clinical picture and diagnosis

Many of those infected are asymptomatic, but adults who accumulate a worm load of 500 or more may be seriously affected. In the early acute phase of heavy infections there is upper abdominal pain, jaundice, tender hepatomegaly, fever and eosinopholia. During the later chronic stages there is recurrent cholangitis, which may lead to fatal septicaemia. The liver becomes firmly enlarged. The development of biliary cirrhosis is marked by generalized pruritus, jaundice and sometimes manifestations of portal hypertension. Clonorchiasis predisposes to chronic biliary carriage of *S. typhi*. If cholangiocarcinoma develops there is rapid deterioration with progressive hepatic enlargement, pain, jaundice and wasting.

The differential diagnosis is similar to that for fascioliasis. (see p. 112)

Treatment

Praziquantel has been effective in doses of 14 mg/kg 3 times daily for 5 days. Bithionol 100 mg/kg is also used orally on alternate days for 2–3 weeks. Hexachlorparaxylene (Hetol) is said to be successful in doses of 100 mg/kg daily for 12 days. In bacterial cholangitis antibiotics such as clindamycin and a cephalosporin in combination are needed. Surgical drainage is needed for biliary obstruction by stones.

Opisthorchis felineus

This is normally a parasite of dogs and cats, but human infections occur not uncommonly in Siberia, India, Japan and East Germany. It is morphologically similar to clonorchis (Fig. 6–1) but can be distinguished from *C. sinesis* by the fact that the testes are posteriorly placed and are compactly shaped bodies. The life-cycle and other features are the same as those of *C. sinensis*.

The pathogenesis, clinical picture and treatment of opisthorchiasis are similar to those of clonorchiasis, but biliary stone formation is apparently rare.

Family Heterophyidae

These are very small, flask-shaped flukes which, in addition to the usual oral and ventral suckers, commonly possess a genital sucker. They are all hermaphrodites. The eggs are operculated and contain a fully developed miracidium when passed.

The adults live in the intestine of man, and of dogs and cats. Only two species, *Heterophyes heterophyes* and *Metagonimus yokogawai*, commonly infect man; but other species may occasionally be parasitic in man.

Heterophyes heterophyes

This worm was first described as a parasite of man in Egypt, but it is very common in Palestine and the Far East, especially China, Japan and the Philippines. The adults occur in the small intestine of man, but more commonly in dogs, cats, wolves and foxes. It is easily recognized, being a minute fluke just visible to the naked eye — about 1.2 mm in length and 0.4 mm in breadth — with the characteristic of the family, the genital sucker, large and prominent. The cuticle is densely covered with spines.

The ova, when seen in the faeces, are almost indistinguishable from those of *Clonorchis sinensis*, and like those of *C. sinensis* contain a fully developed miracidium. The life-cycle is similar to that of *Clonorchis*. The larval forms develop in freshwater snails of the genus *Pironella* or *Cerithidea*, and the cercariae encyst in various species of freshwater fish, especially mullet.

Medical aspects of heterophyiasis

Pathogenesis and clinical features

These small worms adhere to the wall of the small intestine, causing inflammation and superficial ulceration. Occasionally ova enter blood vessels in the intestinal wall and may embolize to the central nervous system and the heart. Egg granulomas in the myocardium and on the mitral valve can result in cardiac failure. Light infections are often asymptomatic. Heavy infections produce upper abdominal pain and diarrhoea.

Treatment

Bephenium hydroxynaphthoate (Alcopar) 5 g daily for 2 days has been used to treat the infestation. Tetrachlorethylene in single doses of 2–3 ml is an alternative.

Metagonimus yokogawai

This parasite is probably very common in the Far East. It is recorded from Japan, China and Russia, and in Europe from Spain and the Balkans. It is very similar morphologically to *H. heterophyes*, but can be distinguished from it by several characteristics:

1. The genital sucker is absent or very poorly developed in *Metagonimus*, and very conspicuous in *Heterophyes*.
2. The ventral sucker is displaced laterally to the right of the ventral line in *Metagonimus*.
3. In *Metagonimus* the genital pore lies in a pit anterior to the ventral sucker, while in *Heterophyes* it lies posterolaterally, in the centre of the genital sucker.

The eggs are indistinguishable from those of *Heterophyes*, and when laid they contain a mature miracidium.

The adult worm lives in the small intestine of man, cats, dogs and pigs. The eggs are passed into water with the faeces of the host, and the first intermediate host is the snail *Semisulcospira*. The second host is a freshwater fish, usually of the genus *Plectoglossus*, in whose flesh the metacercariae encyst. Infection of the definitive host occurs when he (or it) eats raw or lightly cooked fish flesh.

Metagonimiasis has intestinal symptoms similar to those produced by *Heterophyes*. Treatment is as for *Heterophyes* infection.

Superfamily Plagiorchioidea

These are all medium-sized, thick, oval worms that occur in the lungs and other tissues of man and certain carnivores. They are all hermaphrodites. The eggs are passed in the sputum and faeces of the host, they are large, broadly-oval and operculated, and when passed they contain a large, unsegmented ovum. *Paragonimus* is the only genus in this superfamily that commonly parasitizes man.

Paragonimus westermani

Paragonimiasis in man is common only in the Far East, chiefly in Japan, China, Korea and Taiwan, but it has been reported from South and North America and it also occurs in the Philippines, India, Malaysia and parts of West Africa. The reservoir hosts for the human infections are the dog and cat, but species of *Paragonimus* very similar to those parasitizing man have been recorded from many different species of carnivores.

In the mammalian host the adult worms usually live in the lungs, but they have been recorded from many other sites such as the spleen and liver. They are usually enclosed, sometimes in pairs, in a fibrous cyst which retains the eggs until the cyst ruptures and releases them into the bronchi. The living worm is often of a split-pea or spoon shape, but when preserved it tends to become spherical. Its length is 1–1.5 cm, and it is about 0.5 cm in breadth and 0.5 cm in thickness (Fig. 6.1). The integument is covered with short, scale-like spines. The worm is generally reddish-brown when first removed from the host, but preserved specimens are often a dirty grey colour. The ventral sucker is near the middle of the body. The excretory vesicle is large and conspicuous, and extends from the posterior towards the anterior end, dividing the body into two halves. The internal organs can be seen only after the worm has been flattened.

The genital pore lies immediately below the ventral sucker, whereas in the trematodes previously described it lies above the sucker. The uterus is a coiled tube lying well to one side of the middle line. The vitellaria lie in a broad band on each side of the body. There are two lobed testes situated in the posterior part of the body.

The eggs, when passed in the sputum or faeces, are yellowish oval bodies about 90 × 50 μm. The egg when laid contains a single large unsegmented ovum (Fig. 6.2).

The eggs of *Paragonimus* develop only when they reach water, and at an optimum temperature of about 25–30°C the miracidium develops and emerges in about 4 weeks. Further development occurs only in snails of the correct genus — mainly *Semisulcospira* and *Brotia* in the Far East, but other molluscan hosts have been recorded in other parts of the world.

In the snail the miracidium loses its cilia and develops into a sporocyst. The sporocyst then produces rediae, which are liberated by rupture of the sporocyst. These rediae spread through the tissues of the snail, and in turn give rise to daughter rediae that are released by rupture of the parent rediae. The daughter rediae give rise to the cercariae, which bore their way through the body of the snail and escape into the water.

Once in the water the cercariae seek their second intermediate host, which in the case of *P. westermani* is a crab (usually *Eriocheir* or *Potamon*) or a crayfish.

The cercariae may be taken in by the feeding-currents, or may penetrate the articulations of the shell of the crustacean. Metacercariae may be found in the heart, the gills or the muscles.

If man swallows the encysted metacercariae in uncooked crayfish or crabs, the immature flukes hatch in the duodenum, penetrate through the gut wall into the peritoneal cavity, and reach the lungs by boring through the diaphragm. In the lungs the larvae become enclosed in a cyst capsule, and reach maturity in about 4 weeks. Although the lungs are the normal final site of these flukes, some of them never reach this destination but become encapsulated (and sometimes destroyed) in such sites as the peritoneum, mesenteric glands, intestinal muscle and brain, where they may give rise to localized symptoms.

Medical aspects of paragonimiasis

Adult worms are found in fibrous cysts secreted by the host in peribronchial situations; the worms are often in pairs and sometimes degenerate. The lung apices are usually spared. Most cysts communicate with bronchi, allowing egress of eggs. Eggs which remain in lung tissue around cysts give rise to granulomas; atelectasis, bronchiectasis, bacterial pneumonia and haemoptysis complicate the infection. The pleural cavity is often involved, causing pleural adhesions, effusions and pneumothoraces. Ectopic worms may remain in the abdominal cavity or migrate to subcutaneous tissue. Worms can also reach the brain, causing symptoms of cerebral tumour, or the spinal cord, causing paraplegia. Cerebral paragonimiasis is a significant neurosurgical problem in some areas of the Far East.

Clinical picture

Some of those infected have minimal symptoms, the worms usually dying within 5 years. Infection may confer some immunity to reinfection.

A proportion of adults accumulate a gradually increasing worm load and develop a clinical picture of chronic inflammatory lung disease. Cough, expectoration of brownish sputum that is sometimes blood-stained, chest pain, dyspnoea, fever, night sweats and weight loss are common symptoms. On examination scattered crepitations may be found on auscultation, and finger clubbing is seen.

Pleural effusion, pneumothorax, bacterial pneumonia and serious haemoptysis are complications. Abdominal paragonimiasis may cause abdominal pain and diarrhoea — epididymo-orchitis has been recorded due to paragonimiasis. Subcutaneous nodules containing adult worms are sometimes found. Cerebral invasion causes symptoms suggestive of a cerebral tumour.

Diagnosis

Chest X-ray may show migratory infiltrations in the early stages. Later there are peribronchial nodules, cysts or ring shadows in mid and lower zones. There may be some increased hilar shadowing. Examination of the sputum is important in differentiation from tuberculosis. Complement fixation tests are useful in diagnosing cerebral paragonimiasis.

Important differential diagnoses are pulmonary tuberculosis, bronchiectasis, fungal infections and lung abscess.

Treatment

Praziquantel 25 mg/kg 3 times daily for 3 days is the specific treatment of choice. Bithionol 40 mg/kg orally for 15 doses on alternate days is an alternative. Cerebral lesions may respond to chemotherapy, but surgery may be needed in addition.

Superfamily Schistosomatoidea

The Schistosomatoidea differ from the other trematodes infecting man in that the sexes are separate and that the adult worms are blood inhabiting, being parasitic in the portal vein and its radicals. The schistosomes may be long-lived worms, having a maximum life-span of 20–30 years, but on average they live for about 3 years.

The males are shorter and stouter than the females (Fig. 6.1) and their lateral margins are folded ventrally to form a 'gynaecophoric canal' in which the female is held. The female is longer than the male and is filiform in shape. The muscular pharynx is absent, and the two intestinal caeca reunite behind the ventral sucker to form a single canal. The position where the caeca reunite is of diagnostic importance, being different in the different species. The number of testes varies from four to nine, and these always lie in the space between the ventral sucker and the spot where the intestinal caeca unite. In the female Laurer's canal is absent, and the gravid uterus contains a few eggs.

The eggs are not operculated, and they have a spine or knob, the position of which differs in the different species. When laid, the egg contains a fully developed miracidium. The cercariae have bifid tails (Fig. 6.2), and penetrate into the definitive host through unbroken skin. There is no encysted metacercaria stage.

Only one genus in the superfamily, *Schistosoma*, infects man; the species differs in different parts of the world.

Schistosoma haematobium

S. haematobium parasitizes man in various parts of Africa and the Middle East, and in some Mediterranean areas.

The adult worms live, *in copulo*, in the pelvic venous plexuses (namely the vesical, prostatic and uterine plexuses of veins) in man, and occasionally in rodents and monkeys. In both sexes the mouth opens into the oesophagus, which extends as far as the ventral sucker; there is no muscular pharynx. As in other trematodes the oesophagus divides at the anterior margin of the ventral sucker (which in the males is larger than the oral sucker). In the males the two branches then unite again about the middle of the body into a common trunk which pursues a wavy course and terminates blindly at the posterior end. The male is 10–15 mm long and has the normal trematode shape, but because the margins are folded to form the gynaecophoric canal it presents a cylindrical appearance (Fig. 6.1). The oral sucker surrounds the mouth and the ventral sucker is near the oral sucker. The gynaecophoric canal extends backwards from the ventral sucker. The integument is covered with small tubercles, and there are small spines on the suckers and in the gynaecophoric canal. The genital pore is close behind the ventral sucker. There are four testes placed closed together just behind the ventral sucker.

The female is cylindrical and thread-like, and is often reddish-black, compared with the colourless male. It is about 2 cm long but only about 250 μm wide (Fig. 6.1). The ends are pointed, the skin is not tuberculated as in the male, and if there are spines on the suckers they are even smaller than those of the male.

The uterus of the gravid female contains 20–30 eggs. The eggs are compact and spindle-shaped, and measure about 140 $\times$ 50 μm (Fig. 6.2). At one pole they bear a short terminal spine. When laid they contain a highly organized miracidium.

Oviposition usually occurs in the small venules of the vesical plexus. The female, held in the gynaecophoric canal of the male, extends its anterior end far into the smallest venules and deposits the eggs longitudinally, one at a time. Each time an egg is laid the female withdraws a short distance, and she then lays another egg immediately behind the first. In this way the venules are filled with eggs pointing backwards, and the worms *in copulo* then migrate to an adjoining venule. The eggs are held in position by the spines and by the contraction of the blood vessels when the parent worm retires. The eggs work their way through the blood vessels and the mucosa of the urinary bladder, and finally emerge into the cavity of the bladder admixed with extravasated blood. They normally escape with the urine, usually at the end of micturition, but occasionally they may be found in the faeces.

The egg does not hatch in the urine, but when the urine is diluted with water the miracidium becomes very active and the egg hatches (probably owing to osmotic effects). The miracidium ruptures the egg shell and escapes into the water, where it has a life of up to 30 hours. The miracidium swims about by means of its cilia until it finds a suitable snail intermediate host, and while swimming it rapidly and repeatedly changes shape. The miracidium has penetration glands, and shows the beginnings of the genital and excretory systems of the adult. The most important intermediate snail hosts are members of the genus *Bulinus*. The miracidium bores into the soft tissues of the snail, and it ultimately makes it way to the digestive gland where it loses its cilia and other organs and becomes a sporocyst. Multiplication of the sporocysts occurs to such an extent that the digestive gland becomes permeated in a few weeks with a mass of delicate, tubular daughter sporocysts. Several weeks after the infection, further multiplication stops and the daughter sporocysts give rise to the forked-tailed cercariae. Unlike other digenetic trematodes parasitic in man, *Schistosoma* produces no rediae at any stage in its life cycle, all multiplication in the snail taking place at the sporocyst stage. The cercariae finally burst from the sporocyst and escape from the snail into the water.

Man becomes infected when he bathes in, wades in, or drinks water containing the cercariae, which penetrate the skin or mucous membranes by means of their glandular secretions. While penetrating the dermis the tails are cast off, and the bodies of the cercariae (now called schistosomulae) penetrate the tissues by means of the secretions and active muscular movements. Finally they reach the venous circulation, either by entering a peripheral venule or via the lymph vessels. From here they are carried through the right side of the heart to the pulmonary capillaries. It requires some days for the larvae to pass through the capillary bed in the lungs, and then they are carried through the left side of the heart into the systemic circulation. From the abdominal aorta some of them enter the mesenteric artery, then they pass through the capillary bed in the intestine and enter the portal circulation. They finally reach the liver about 5 days after penetration. Inside the liver (still in the blood vessels) they grow into adults in about another 2 weeks. After becoming sexually differentiated they move out of the liver against the blood current, migrating into the inferior mesenteric vein and eventually into the vesical and pelvic plexuses. The worms reach their final site 1–3 months after the cercariae penetrate the skin. The females commence laying eggs soon after their arrival in the plexuses.

Schistosoma mansoni

This parasite occurs widely in Africa, in South America, and in the Caribbean. The adults live in the plexuses in the colonic and rectal areas, and also in the branches of the portal vein in the liver. *S. mansoni* is also a parasite of some rodents and monkeys.

The morphology is essentially the same as that of *S. haematobium*. The male is slightly smaller than that of *S. haematobium*, being only 1 cm long. After the primary bifurcation of the alimentary canal, the two caeca reunite in the upper half of the body. The common caecum then usually bifurcates again, and the branches later reunite again. Behind the ventral sucker the integument is covered with tubercles that are much bigger than those of *S. haematobium*. The genital system is similar to that of *S. haematobium* except that there are eight or nine testes arranged in a zigzag row. The female too, is small, being only 1.4 cm long. The ovary is anterior to the middle of the body, but otherwise the genital system is similar to that of *S. haematobium*. The gravid uterus contains only up to three eggs, usually one one.

The eggs are bluntly oval, the same size as those of *S. haematobium* (about $150 \times 60 \, \mu m$). and have a lateral spine (Fig. 6.2). The miracidium, sporocyst and cercaria are similar to those of *S. haematobium*. The eggs are passed in faeces (rarely in urine) and the miracidium hatches when the egg gets into water. The miracidium enters snails of the genus *Biomphalaria* or *Tropicorbis*, and the subsequent development in the snail is similar to that of *S. haematobium*. The cercaria, after escaping from the snail, has a maximum life of about 30 hours. As in *S. haematobium*, the cercariae stick to the skin of the bather or wader by means of their ventral suckers, and as the water begins to evoporate the cercariae penetrate the skin. The schistosomulae are carried to the liver by the same route as those of *S. haematobium*. Their subsequent behaviour differs slightly from that of *S. haematobium*; they migrate against the blood stream into the inferior mesenteric vein and reach the capillaries of the sigmoidorectal area where the eggs are laid. The eggs then make their way through into the rectum and pass out with the faeces. In some cases, where the adult worms are in the vesical plexuses, eggs may be passed with the urine.

Schistosoma japonicum

This is a parasite of the Far East, being found in China, Japan, Taiwan, Burma and the Philippines. It occurs not only in man but also in horses, cattle, pigs, rodents, cats and dogs.

The morphology is basically the same as that of the other schistosomes. The male measures just over 1 cm in length, but unlike in the other species of *Schistosoma* parasitic in man the integument is smooth. After the primary bifurcation of the alimentary canal, the two caeca reunite at a point about three-quarters of the length of the worm from the anterior end. The common trunk then pursues a wavy course to the end of the body, where it terminates blindly. There are between six and eight testes, arranged in a single file, but otherwise the organs are as in the other species. The female is about 2 cm in length. The ovary is situated near the middle of the body and the vitelline glands occupy the posterior half. The gravid uterus always contains more than 50 eggs, and may contain up to 100.

The eggs are distinctly smaller than those of the other two species, measuring 90×50 μm (Fig. 6.2). They have a minute hook or knob near one pole and at the side. They are passed only in the faeces, and contain fully developed miracidia. After the eggs are passed the miracidium hatches in the water. The miracidium is similar to those of the other species, and develops further in snails of the genus *Oncomelania*. The sporocysts and cercariae are similar to those of the other species. After penetrating the skin of man the cercariae lose their tails, and the schistosomulae are carried to the liver. They grow into adult worms and become sexually mature in the portal veins in the liver, then migrate against the blood stream into the superior mesenteric veins and finally reach the capillaries of the small intestine. Thus *S. japonicum* settles in the superior and inferior mesenteric vein and their capillaries, while the other species settle mainly in the inferior mesenteric veins and its capillaries. The eggs of *S. japonicum* finally ulcerate their way through the walls of the blood vessels and the mucosa of the intestine, and escape with the faeces.

Schistosoma infections (schistosomiasis)

Pathogenesis

The pathogenesis of schistosomiasis is complicated, and results from the host's immune reactions to the adult and developing worms and their products, particularly the eggs. The most serious lesions arise from cell-mediated immune granulomas and immune complex reactions surrounding eggs that have been arrested in the tissues near the bowel and bladder, or in the liver and lungs. The liver, lungs and nervous system become involved when eggs fail to penetrate the local vein wall on their way to the exterior and are carried by the blood stream to other areas. About 50 per cent of eggs fail to reach the exterior. Many granulomas probably resolve, but some heal with fibrosis causing distortion of tissues, such as strictures of the ureters.

The extent of the damage caused depends on the species of schistosome, the worm load, the duration of infection, and possibly individual immune reactivity. The distribution of worm loads in a population is uneven; most have a small load of ten pairs or less, but a few have a much heavier load. The latter are likely to suffer significant damage and be potent sources of snail infections. The outcome of infection may partly depend on the extent of the initial cercarial exposure. If massive early exposure takes place, large numbers of adult worms may establish themselves before concomitant immunity is gained, and rein-fection and worm load are limited.

Other pathological effects include a local reaction to schistosomules on skin penetration and an immune complex febrile illness 4–6 weeks after infection. This illness is more likely in *S. japonicum* and *S. mansoni* infections with a heavy cercarial exposure. Other processes that cause damage include wandering eggs reaching the genitalia and other organs; anaemia; immune complex nephritis; recurrent *Salmonella* infections; and carcinogenesis.

The pathology of schistosomiasis is summarized in Table 6.1.

Immunity to schistosomiasis

Much experimental work on immunity to schistosomiasis has been carried out in animals. In man there is little protective immunity against adult worms, which may live 20 years or longer although 2–4 years is a more usual life-span. Adult worms protect themselves against host immune processes by including host antigenic material in their integument and presumably not being recognized as 'foreign' by immunocytes. In endemic areas community infection tends to peak around adolescence and then slowly declines.

Clinical aspects

Most schistosomal infections are light, and the majority of those infected do not suffer serious permanent damage. There is controversy about the extent of serious disease as a result of *S. haematobium* infections. In areas of heavy trans-mission such as Egypt and the Republic of Sudan, schistosomiasis is a serious public health problem. In general *S. japonicum* is the most serious variety of schistosomiasis, and this pathogenicity is related to its high egg output.

Medical aspects of schistosomiasis mansoni

'Bather's itch' is an itchy papular rash lasting a few days after cercarial invasion. It occurs only in some of those already sensitized to cercariae, and can be alle-viated by antihistamine drugs. Sometimes, soon after heavy cercarial invasion, there is a mild febrile illness lasting about a week, coincident with the passage of schistosomules to the portal vein via the lungs.

In some heavily infected patients there is a more serious febrile illness beginning 4–6 weeks after infection and lasting 2–8 weeks; this is known as Katayama fever, being first described in *S. japonicum* infections. Katayama fever occurs during worm maturation and early egg deposition, and results from an immune complex reaction to developing worms, their secretions, and eggs reaching the liver. Katayama fever resembles serum sickness; features include fever, abdominal pain, diarrhoea, cough, urticaria, hepatosplenomegaly, gene-ralized lymphadenopathy and eosinophilia. Serological tests for schistosomiasis are positive, but eggs are not found in the stools at this stage. Usually the febrile

Table 6.1 Pathogenesis of schistosomiasis

Stage	Pathological process	Results	Comments
Early invasion	Immediate and delayed reaction to schistosomules	*Papular, itchy skin rash* lasting a few days; occasional mild systemic illness during early migration — lasts 1–2 weeks; 'Bathers' itch'	Often not seen; not serious; similar skin rash commonly due to non-maturing animal and bird schistosomules
Intermediate stage beginning 4–6 weeks after infection and during egg laying	Immune complex reaction to developing worms, their secretions and early egg laying	*Febrile illness like serum sickness* lasting up to 8 weeks; fever, abdominal pain, diarrhoea, hepatosplenomegaly, lymphadenopathy, urticaria and eosinophilia; 'Katayama fever'	Seen particularly in S. *japonicum* and less so in S. *mansoni* after heavy infection; rarely fatal
	Arrest of eggs in tissues; CMI, granulomas	*Granuloma formation in submucosa of colon* (mansoni, japonicum); ileum (japonicum) *urinary tract* (haematobium) cause ulceration bleeding and polyps in bowel and bladder	*Main pathological process;* granulomas favourably affected by chemotherapy, e.g. ureteric blockage may be reversed
	Passage of eggs through mucosa of bladder and bowel	Relatively minor damage to *mucosa of* bladder and bowel; some bleeding	Responsible for some blood in urine and stools
	Ectopic egg passage in venous circulation	Passage to liver — endophlebitis and blockage of portal radicles causes *presinusoidal portal hypertension*	*Causes GIT bleeding* (S. mansoni *and* S. japonicum) — leading cause of *death*
		Passage to lungs — endophlebitis and block of pulmonary arterioles causes pulmonary hypertension	Usually in S.*m.* and S.*j.* after liver involvement, sometimes in S. *haematobium*
		Passage to brain — local granuloma	S. *japonicum* — causes epilepsy and encephalopathy
		Passage to spinal cord — local granuloma	S. *mansoni* — causes paraplegia
	'Wandering' tissue ova	Ova may reach genitalia and surrounding skin in S. *haematobium*, causing	In S. *haematobium*, involvement of cervix not uncommon

Table 6.1—*cont'd*

Stage	Pathological process	Results	Comments
		granulomata on penis, cervix fallopian tubes; rarely pelvic lympthatic blockage with genital elephantiasis Serosal surface of intestine and peritoneum may be involved	*S. japonicum, S. mansoni* may cause intestinal adhesions
	Red cell destruction and loss	Anaemia due to GIT and urinary bleeding; hypersplenism in portal hypertension and some autoimmune haemolysis	Anaemia not usually severe except after portal hypertension; GIT bleeding
Late	Fibrotic healing of granulomas	Fibrotic stricture of ureters — *hydronephrosis and renal failure* *Fibrosis of bladder* Fibrosis of colonic wall	Main cause of death in *S. haematobium* Disabling urinary frequency May cause abdominal pains; rarely intestinal obstruction
	Carcinogenesis	*Late carcinoma bladder (squamous)* Possible carcinoma of colon Organisms may be protected from host immunity and chemotherapy on the surface or in the gut of schistosomes	*S. haematobium* *S. japonicum*
	Chronic low grade Salmonella septicaemia		
	Immune complex nephritis	Nephrotic syndrome in *S. mansoni* and *S. haematobium*	Probably not uncommon

illness gradually resolves, but deaths have been recorded in *S. japonicum* Katayama fever.

When egg laying is established some patients have abdominal pain and diarrhoea with or without blood, but many have no abdominal symptoms. There may be some splenic enlargement not, at this stage, due to portal hypertension. Abdominal pain and diarrhoea often subside in 6–12 months, but those with heavy infection may have troublesome chronic abdominal pain with palpable colonic masses and rarely even intestinal obstruction.

Complications

Portal hypertension

Bleeding oesophageal varices secondary to portal hypertension are the commonest cause of death in *S. mansoni* and *S. japonicum* infections. Presinusoidal portal hypertension develops in a proportion after years of infection. Embolisation of eggs to small portal vessels causes endophlebitis and surrounding granuloma formation with ultimate fibrous vascular obstruction. The condition is known as 'pipestem fibrosis' with fibrotic changes around portal tracts, some arterial neovascularization of the damaged areas but with reasonable preservation of liver function. Initially the liver enlarges, later it shrinks; the spleen enlarges and hypersplenism with anaemia develops. Recurrent severe haemorrhage from oesophageal varices is the most serious effect. Ascites, oedema and jaundice are late symptoms, occurring if liver failure develops. People with schistosomiasis have difficulty in clearing their serum of hepatitis B surface antigen — a common infection in the tropics — and this may contribute to hepatic failure in schistosomiasis.

Pulmonary hypertension

When portal-systemic venous anastamoses are present following portal hypertension, ectopic eggs may reach the pulmonary arterioles causing blockage and pulmonary hypertension. The patient has the usual symptoms and signs of cor pulmonale with dyspnoea, enlarged right ventricle, loud pulmonary second sound, right-sided failure, enlarged pulmonary conus visible radiologically, and ECG right ventricular hypertrophy. The condition is irreversible.

Neurological schistosomiasis

Ectopic eggs may cause granulomas in the CNS causing focal damage. Aberrant worms can reach the CNS and lay eggs there. Usually in *S. mansoni* infections neurological lesions are in the spinal cord causing paraglegia or cauda equina lesions. There may be a favourable response to chemotherapy.

Anaemia

Anaemia is sometimes marked; GIT haemorrhage, hypersplenism and a mild autoimmune haemolysis are contributory factors.

Other complications

Extensive schistosomal polyposis causes chronic diarrhoea, a protein-losing enteropathy and tenesmus. A clinical picture resembling malabsorption results.

Fibrous scarring leading to intestinal obstruction is an unusual complication. Nephrotic syndrome due to immune complex nephritis has been described, and is more common in those with chronic *Salmonella* infection associated with schistosomiasis.

Clinical diagnosis

The differential diagnosis depends on the stage of the disease. Katayama fever may be confused with other causes of prolonged fever, such as typhoid and tuberculosis. Eosinophilia and positive serological tests for schistosomiasis are helpful diagnostically, but eggs are not present in the stools. Antischistosome drugs are not curative at this stage, but corticosteroids are used in severe cases. The dysenteric phase needs differentiation from amoebic dysentery and ulcerative colitis. Hepatic schistosomasis should be distinguished from other causes of hepatosplenomegaly and portal hypertension, including portal cirrhosis, tropical splenomegaly, visceral leishmaniasis and lymphoma.

Treatment

Subjects passing viable eggs in the stools and cases with suspected neurological lesions should be treated. The objective is to reduce the worm load to such low levels that serious harm does not occur. Repeated courses of treatment in an effort to eliminate the infection completely may expose the patient to the toxic effects of drugs, although this is less of a problem with modern drugs than it was formerly. Complete eradication of infection may theoretically interfere with concomitant immunity, which may be protective in those who continue to be exposed to infection.

The specific drugs of choice are oxamniquine and praziquantel. Oxamniquine is a tetrahydroquinoline given orally; the intramuscular preparations caused local pain. Toxic symptoms are mild temporary giddiness and fever. The dosage of 15 mg/kg on two successive nights achieves a high cure rate in many areas, but in Zimbabwe, Egypt and the Sudan double this dose is recommended. Praziquantel is effective when given orally in all three varieties of schistosomiasis, and has low toxicity. The dose is 50 mg/kg in one dose. Oxamniquine and praziquantel can safely be given to patients with liver involvement.

Niridazole (a nitrothiazole) is in wide use. It is given orally in doses of 25 mg/kg body weight daily for 7 days, the drug being given in three daily divided doses. It is sometimes toxic, causing vomiting, headache, fits, mental changes and even fatal coma. Niridazole should not be given to people with liver disease or a history of epilepsy.

Antimonial drugs are now obsolete.

Supportive and surgical treatment

Transfusion is needed after gastrointestinal bleeding. Portal hypertension can be relieved by splenectomy and lienorenal shunt if liver function is still good. Colonic polypectomy via a fibre-optic colonoscope has been used with benefit in multiple polyposis.

Medical aspects of schistosomiasis japonicum

Pathogenesis and clinical manifestations

These are generally similar to those of *S. mansoni*, but the ileum is involved as well as the colon. Because of the greater egg production the disease is more severe, sometimes proceeding to a fatal termination within 5 years with portal hypertension and cachexia. The Katayama fever syndrome is more common and severe than in *S. mansoni* infections, and cerebral neurological lesions are more frequent.

Treatment

S. japonicum is more resistant to chemotherapy than is *S. mansoni* or *S. haematobium*. Praziquantel is the drug of choice, used as described above for *S. mansoni*.

Formerly sodium antimony tartrate or 'tartar emetic' were used, but these were toxic.

Medical aspects of schistosomiasis haematobium

Clinical manifestations

Many of those infected are asymptomatic or mildly affected. Some will have urinary symptoms such as terminal haematuria and suprapubic, urethral or perineal pain for months or years during childhood and adolescence. Generally the symptoms gradually abate spontaneously and no serious harm is done, although eggs continue to be excreted in diminishing numbers in the urine. In some of those with heavy infections serious complications supervene. Fibrosis of the bladder may lead to reduced capacity, disabling urinary frequency, and painful micturition. There may be vesical stone formation, papillomata in the bladder, and recurrent urinary bacterial infection. There is a considerable increase in the incidence of squamous cell bladder cancer in those with *S. haematobium* infection, and this gives rise to renewed and considerable haematuria.

Hydronephrosis due to ureteric blockage by granulomata is reversible with chemotherapy, which is worth trying before resorting to surgery; surgery is necessary for fibrous stricture. Ultimately an uncertain but small proportion of those infected die of renal failure due to obstructive uropathy. Eggs may reach the urethral mucosa, and urethral stricture, sometimes with perineal fistulae, results. Granulomatous lesions may be found on the penis, and in the prostate, cervix and fallopian tubes. Schistosomiasis predisposes to chronic urinary excretion of *S. typhi*, and patients may have recurrent *Salmonella* bacteraemia. The organisms shelter in or on the adult schistosomes, gaining protection from immune destruction.

Schistosomiasis is a common cause of calcification of the bladder, seen radiologically. The calcium is laid down in subepithelial eggs and granulomas, and may gradually disappear in the course of years.

Clinical diagnosis

S. haematobium is the commonest cause of haematuria (classically terminal) in endemic areas. Many asymptomatic people excrete a few eggs, and their presence does not necessarily incriminate schistosomiasis as the cause of bleeding. Monitoring response to treatment, careful follow-up and sometimes cystoscopy are necessary. In schistosomiasis cystoscopy shows 'sandy patches' of abnormal mucosa and sometimes papillomata. Urinary stone, tumour, tuberculosis and sickle-cell disease and trait may cause haematuria in the tropics and indeed coexist with schistosomiasis. IVP is needed to demonstrate ureteric obstruction.

Treatment

Metrifonate, an organophosphorus anticholinesterase drug, is given orally in two doses of 10 mg/kg with a 2-week interval. Toxic side effects are unusual, although abdominal cramps, vomiting and diarrhoea may be seen. The red blood cell cholinesterase is markedly depressed for 2 weeks after dosage; and contact with organophosphate insecticides should be avoided during this time.

Niridazole is used as for *S. mansoni* infection. A single dose of metrifonate 12.5 mg/kg together with niridazole 500 mg has also proved effective. Praziquantel is also effective.

Surgical treatment is needed to relieve fibrous ureteric stricture, and operations have also been carried out to increase the capacities of fibrosed bladders using portions of ileum.

Laboratory identification of trematodes

Human infections with trematodes are usually identified by finding characteristic eggs in the faeces, or more rarely in the urine or sputum. Only very occasionally are adult worms passed out from the body, and in these cases identifiable eggs will almost certainly be found as well. Immunofluorescence tests have also proved useful for diagnosis.

Identification of eggs

In general, the eggs of the common trematode parasites of man (Fig. 6.2) are readily identifiable, although there may be difficulty in distinguishing between the eggs of different members of the '*Clonorchis* group' of worms.

Fasciolopsis buski eggs (see Fig. 9.2)

The eggs vary considerably in size and form, but on average are ovoid, about 135 μm long and 85 μm wide. They are yellowish-brown, and have an operculum that is difficult to see in freshly passed eggs. When freshly passed the egg contains a fertilized undeveloped ovum surrounded by yolk cells.

Fasciola hepatica eggs (see Fig 9.2)

The eggs are very similar to those of *F. buski,* and differentiation of the two species of eggs is not practicable. *F. hepatica* is essentially a parasite of herbivores, but human infections have been reported from many parts of the world, and in some countries. *F. hepatica* has become of definite public health importance.

Clonorchis sinensis eggs (see Fig. 9.2)

The eggs are yellowish-brown, shaped rather like an old-fashioned electric light bulb, and about 30 μm long and 15 μm wide. The operculum is convex and easily seen because of the thickened collar; and there is frequently a small knob-like extension at the end of the shell opposite the operculum. The egg contains a fully developed miracidium when laid (see note under *Heterophyes*).

Opisthorchis felineus eggs

The eggs are yellowish-brown, an elongated ovoid in shape, and about 30 μm long and 11 μm wide. The operculum fits closely into the thickened rim of the shell, so that there is a conspicuous collar; and there may be a minute knob-like extension at the end of the shell opposite to the operculum. The egg contains a fully developed miracidium when laid (see note under *Heterophyes*).

Heterophyes heterophyes eggs

The eggs are yellowish-brown, ovoid, and about 28 μm long and 16 μm wide. The operculum is rather pointed, and there is only a very slight thickening of the rim of the shell. The egg contains a fully developed miracidium when laid.
NOTE: The eggs of the *Metagonimus yokogawai* are very similar to those of *Heterophyes.* Some morphological differences have been described — for example that the operculum of *Metagonimus* is rounded and not pointed — but the differences are too slight to be of practical importance. The eggs of *Clonorchis* and *Opisthorchis* are also very easily confused with those of the two heterophid worms. Although the eggs of *Opisthorchis* usually appear narrow, and those of *Clonorchis* may (at the extreme end of their size range) be as large as 35 × 19 μm, the size ranges of the four species overlap. And as helminth eggs generally show considerable morphological variation within a species, differentiation of these four species of eggs is difficult.

Paragonimus westermani eggs (see Fig. 9.2)

The eggs are yellowish-brown, ovoid, and about 100 μm long and 55 μm wide. The operculum is rather flattened, and is easily seen because of the thickened collar. When passed the egg contains a large unsegmented ovum. The eggs are most commonly found in the sputum, but sometimes occur in the faeces.

Schistosoma haematobium eggs (see Fig. 9.2)

The eggs are light yellowish-brown, spindle shaped, and about 140 μm long and 50 μm wide. At one end is a distinct terminal spine. When passed the egg contains a fully developed miracidium. The eggs are normally passed in the urine, usually at the end of the micturition, but they may occasionally be passed in the faeces.

Schistosoma mansoni eggs (see Fig. 9.2)

The eggs are light yellowish-brown, ovoid, and about 150 μm long and 60 μm wide. The egg has a large lateral spine, shaped like a rose thorn, towards one end. When passed the egg contains a fully developed miracidium. The eggs are normally passed in the faeces, but may rarely be found in the urine.

Schistosoma japonicum eggs (see Fig. 9.2)

The eggs are paler in colour and distinctly rounder than those of the other schistosomes parasitic in man, and measure about 90 μm long and 70 μm wide. Near one end of the egg is a small lateral spine or knob, which is often very difficult to see. When passed the egg contains a fully developed miracidium. The eggs are passed in the faeces.

Control of schistosomiasis

Over 200 million people are infected with schistosomiasis, and this number is increasing with extension of irrigation schemes which often result in spread of the disease. Schistosomiasis is a serious public health problem in Africa, South America and Asia. When irrigation schemes or man-made lakes are planned, the possibility of schistosomiasis must be considered and measures taken to make the water an unsuitable habitat for the snail vectors and to prevent the introduction of infection.

Mathematical models have been created to assess the relative importance of various strategies of prevention. It is considered that prevention of contamination of water by schistosome eggs would be difficult and would not be a very effective preventive measure because of the enormous multiplication of the parasites within snails. Destruction of vector snails and mass treatment of schistosome egg excretors should be the most effective control measures. Animal reservoirs are of little importance in *S. haematobium* or *S. mansoni* infections, but are very important in the case of *S. japonicum*. Animal reservoirs and the amphibious nature of the vector snails make control of *S. japonicum* very difficult, but control seems to have succeeded in China.

Control of schistosomiasis is far from easy, and is expensive. Many schemes have failed, and a combination of methods is needed. Principles of control are outlined in Table 6.2.

General principles of trematode control

Infections depend on a chain of events, namely contamination of water by infected excreta of animals or man: infection of freshwater snails by miracidia; infection of fish, crustacea or water plants by cercariae: and finally, con-

Table 6.2 Principles of control of schistosomiasis

Theoretical control measures	Practical control measures	Comments
Prevention of contamination of water sources with schistosome eggs	Provision (and use of) latrines; siting of villages away from water supplies; health education	Difficult to achieve
Destruction of miracidia	Molluscicides may have some action	
Elimination of vector snail population	1. Make habitats unsuitable for snails; increase flow of water; remove vegetation; cover irrigation channels; use intermittent irrigation with drying-out periods.	
	2. Application of chemical molluscicides, e.g. frescon is often very effective	Offensive to ecologists; may poison fish; costly
	3. Biological control by snail predators	So far not very effective
Prevent contact of humans with cercariae	Provide piped water supply	Most important for general disease control
	Provide clean bathing sites; footbridges over canals; (?) cercarial destruction; protective clothing has little practical application	
Eliminate reservoir of infection (mainly infected children and adolescents)	Mass chemotherapy; targeted chemotherapy of children and adolescents	Safe oral drugs now available; repeated treatment may be needed
Protection of recipients by vaccination	Vaccine not available yet	Vaccination had some effect in animals

sumption by man of metacercariae in fish, in crustacea, on plants, or by direct contamination of fingers. Possible points of intervention in the transmission cycle can be considered.

The infections are usually zoonotic, so prevention of contamination of the freshwater habitats of the snail intermediate hosts is not possible. Improved sanitation, however, would reduce the chances of contamination by human excreta. On the other hand, fish is a valuable source of protein and so human and animal excreta may deliberately be put into fish ponds to increase the yield of fish.

Destruction of the vector snail populations is impracticable. The best hope for prevention lies in the proper preparation of fish, crustacea and water plants for human consumption. Raw, undercooked or pickled fish is a delicacy in many areas, crustacea may be eaten raw or steeped in wine, and raw crayfish juice is used as a cure for diarrhoea. People at risk should be made aware of the necessity to cook fish and crustacea adequately, and to wash their hands after handling them. Water plants should not be peeled with the teeth. In order to prevent fascioliasis, watercress should be used for human consumption only after collection from safe, uncontaminated water sources.

Mass treatment would reduce worm loads in individuals, but it is not a satisfactory means of control where there are animal reservoirs. Mass treatment has, however, been proposed as a means of control of paragonimiasis in Japan, where man is considered to be the main reservoir of infection.

Further reading

Ashford RW, Hall AJ, Babona D. Distribution and abundance of intestinal helminths in man in western Papua New Guinea with special reference to *Strongyloides*. *Ann Trop Med Parasitol* 1984: **75**: 269–79.

Hardman EW, Jones RLH, Davies AH. Fascioliasis — a large outbreak. *Brit Med Journal* 1970; **3**: 502–05.

Jordan P, Webbe G. *Schistosomiasis: Epidemiology, Treatment and Control*. London: Heinemann, 1982.

Komiya Y. *Clonorchis* and clonorchiasis. *Adv Parasitol* 1966: **4**: 53–106.

Koompirochana C, Sonakul D, Chinda K *et al*. Opisthorchiasis: a clinicopathological study of 154 autopsy cases. Asian J Trop Med Pub Hlth 1978; **9**: 60–64.

Mahmoud AAF. Schistosomiasis. In: Warren KS and Mahmoud AAF (eds) *Tropical and Geographical Medicine* New York: McGraw-Hill 1984 443–57.

Nwokolo C. Endemic paragonimiasis in Eastern Nigeria. *Trop Geograph Med* 1972 **24**: 138–47.

Rahman KM, Idris M, Azad Khan AK. A study of fasiolopsiasis in Bangladesh. *J Trop Med Hyg* 1981; **84**: 81–6

Seah SKK. Digenetic trematodes *Clin Gastroenterol* 1978; **7**: 87–104.

Sheir ZM, El-Shabrawy AEM. Demographic, clinical and therapeutic appraisal of heterophyiasis. *J Trop Med Hyg* 970; **73**: 148–52.

Warren KS. The pathology, pathobiology and pathogenesis of schistosomiasis. *Nature*, London 1978; **273**: 609–12.

Warren KS. Schistosomiasis. In: Weatherall DJ, Ledingham JGG and Warrell DA (eds) *Oxford Textbook of Medicine* Vol. 5. Oxford; University Press, 1983 449–55.

WHO *Epidemiology and Control of Schistosomiasis*. Geneva; WHO Technical Report Series **643**, 1980.

Yokogawa M. *Paragonimus* and paragonimiasis. *Adv Parasitol* 1969; **7**: 375–87.

7

The roundworms

The roundworms, or nematodes, are a large group of worms of comparatively simple organization, nearly all of which are strangers to everyone but zoologists even though they play an extremely important role in nature. They have been able to exploit nearly every conceivable terrestrial and aquatic habitat. Most plants are parasitized by nematodes, and probably every animal species harbours some nematode parasite. Only about a dozen species are important human parasites, although over 50 species have been found in man on occasions. Most of the free-living nematodes, and most of those parasitic in invertebrates and plants, are so small and transparent as to be scarcely visible to the naked eye. These forms have a very simple life-cycle. The species parasitic in vertebrates are relative giants, some up to several feet in length, and may have much more complicated life-cycles.

The typical nematode is an elongated, cylindrical worm without any appendages, tapering more or less at each end, and enclosed in a very tough and impermeable transparent or semitransparent cuticle. Usually the cuticle is marked externally by fine transverse striations, and there may be bristles, spines, ridges or expansions of various kinds. In some parasitic forms there are fin-like expansions in the neck region of both sexes (cervical alae) or in the tail region of males (caudal alae).

The mouth may be rounded or slit-like, and is often provided anteriorly with lips. It sometimes leads to a large buccal cavity lined wtih chitin, which may bear cutting organs in the shape of teeth or plates or both. In other cases the buccal cavity is extremely small, and the mouth is just the termination of the oesophagus. The buccal cavity leads into the alimentary canal, which consists of oesophagus and intestine and ends in a subterminal anus. The intestine is a flat or cylindrical tube, usually straight, and is lined with a single layer of cells. At the posterior end there is a chitinized rectum. In the female the intestine has an anal opening separate from the reproductive system, but in the male the intestine and the reproductive system open into a common cloaca.

With rare exceptions the parasitic nematodes have separate sexes that are externally indistinguishable, except that usually the males are smaller than the females and the form of the tail differs in the two sexes. In both sexes the reproductive system consists primarily of long tubules, part of which serve as ovaries or testes and part as ducts. In all parasitic nematodes the male system is reduced to a single tubule, but (with rare exceptions) the female system is double, and in a few species is further redoubled.

The development of the nematodes is a comparatively simple process. The original egg cell, after being enclosed in a membrane or shell, divides by simple fission until it forms a solid morula, which then assumes a 'tadpole' shape and becomes hollow inside. This larva then develops into an elongated embryo with a simple digestive tract, which after some further growth forms the definitive first larval stage. Thereafter the development proceeds slowly, and it is punctuated by a series of moults, usually four. However, in some nematodes one or two of the moults may occur in the egg before hatching. The successive larval instars may differ in details of structure, but they are never totally unlike each other.

The stage of development at the time the eggs are laid varies greatly, eggs of different species apparently being dependent on different oxygen requirements for development. Some leave the female's body unsegmented (e.g. *Ascaris* and *Trichuris*), some in the early stages of segmentation (e.g. hookworms), and some in the tadpole stage (e.g. *Enterobius*). All these species lay incompletely developed eggs, and the nematode is said to be oviparous. Other species (e.g. *Strongyloides)* lay eggs containing fully developed embryos that hatch immediately, and these species are said to be ovo-viviparous. Finally, some nematodes (e.g. *Trichinella* and the filarias) produce larvae, not eggs, and these species are said to be viviparous.

Usually no further development occurs until the eggs or embryos have reached a new environment, either outside the body or in an intermediate host; an exception is *Trichinella*, whose embryos find their new environment in the muscles of the parental host. In the new environment the embryo, either inside the egg or after hatching from it, commonly undergoes two more moults and becomes a third-stage larva before it is infective to another definitive host. When it has reached this third stage it ceases to grow or develop until transfer to a new definitive host is accomplished.

The simplest type of life-cycle is that in which embryonated eggs are swallowed by the host. The embryos, usually in their third stage, hatch in the intestine and may either develop there, burying themselves temporarily in the mucous membrane (e.g. *Enterobius* or *Trichuris*), or they may make a preliminary journey through the host's body and back to the intestine (e.g. *Ascaris*). This simple cycle may be modified by the first-stage larva hatching outside the body, developing to the third stage as a free-living form, and then re-entering the definitive host either by burrowing through the skin (e.g. hookworms) or being swallowed with vegetation (e.g. *Haemonchus*). *Trichinella* produces embryos that encyst in the host muscles and wait to be eaten by another host, thus substituting the original host for the outside world as a place for preliminary partial development. The filariae substitute insects and other invertebrates as a place for partial development, thus requiring a true intermediate host. A few nematodes (e.g. *Gnathostoma*) require two intermediate hosts; the gnathostome larva develops first in *Cyclops*, then in a fish or other cold-blooded vertebrate, and finally reaches sexual maturity in a mammal. Some nematodes, after having reached the infective stage, can re-encyst if they get into an unsuitable host. The methods of escaping from and of re-entering the correct final host vary, different species having different modifications in the life-cycle.

The parasitic nematodes have undoubtedly evolved from several families of free-living nematodes, and so cannot be classified separately from the free-living forms. There is no general agreement on the classification of the nematodes, partly because many new species are still being named; but fortunately there is no confusion over specific names, even though different authorities may refer the same genus to different taxonomic groups. The nematodes

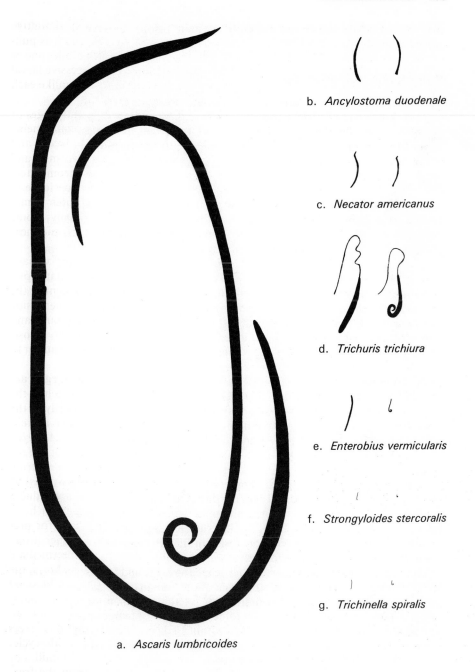

b. *Ancylostoma duodenale*

c. *Necator americanus*

d. *Trichuris trichiura*

e. *Enterobius vermicularis*

f. *Strongyloides stercoralis*

g. *Trichinella spiralis*

a. *Ascaris lumbricoides*

Fig. 7.1 Actual sizes of common Nematode parasites of Man. For all species, the female worm is shown on the left and the male worm on the right.

that in the adult stages are parasitic in man belong to several so-called superfamilies.

Superfamily Ascaridoidea

These are stout worms of large size. The mouth possesses three lips, one dorsal and two lateroventral. The oesophagus is muscular and club-shaped, without a posterior bulb. The females are not much larger than the males. The males possess two spicules, and the tail of the male is curved ventrally.

Ascaris lumbricoides

A. lumbricoides is a well-known parasite, but the important details of its life-cycle were unknown before 1916, and the factors influencing its epidemiology were not elucidated until after 1930. This is probably because, in general, *Ascaris* infections were not thought to be serious — but early in the present century the worm became recognized as an injurious and sometimes dangerous parasite.

   A. lumbricoides is the largest intestinal nematode parasitizing man, and resembles the earthworm. When fresh from the intestine it is light brown or pink in colour, but it gradually turns white. It is rounded in section and tapering at both ends, the anterior end being thinner than the posterior. The male is about 15–25 cm long, and the female is 25–35 cm long. The mouth is guarded by three lips, one dorsal and two lateroventral, each with minute papillae. The male can be distinguished by its curled pointed tail, which is armed with two spicules. The female has a straight blunt tail. (Fig. 7.1)

   The worm passes its life-cycle in one species of host, and no intermediate host is required, although there is a free-living period to allow transference from one host to another. The adult lives in the small intestine where it is said to feed on the semidigested food of the host, but there is evidence that it commonly attaches to the mucous membrane with its lips and sucks blood and tissue juices. The female produces a very great number of eggs, and it has been estimated that one female will produce 200 000 eggs per day. The eggs have a thick, clear inner shell usually covered over by a warty albuminous coat which is stained yellow or brown in the intestine (Fig. 7.2). Within the clear egg shell is a very delicate vitelline membrane that is even more resistant than the egg shell, and as a result some eggs can remain viable for years.

   The eggs are unsegmented when they leave the host, and in order to develop they require a temperature lower than that of the human body, at least a trace of moisture, and oxygen. Complete desiccation is lethal, but in moist soil they may remain viable for years. Under favourable conditions of temperature, moisture and air the eggs develop active embryos within 14 days. These larvae, however, are not infective until they have developed further and moulted to the second stage, which requires an extra week or two.

   When the eggs are swallowed by man they pass through the stomach and the larvae hatch in the small intestine. The larvae measure about 25 μm in length. They penetrate the wall of the intestine and are carried by the portal circulation to the liver, then via the right side of the heart to the lungs. In the alveolar walls of the lungs they moult twice (first on the fifth day and second on the tenth day)

Egg of
Ascaris lumbricoides

Egg of
Enterobius vermicularis

Egg of
Ancylostoma or *Necator*

Egg of
Trichuris trichiura

Egg of
Capillaria philippinensis

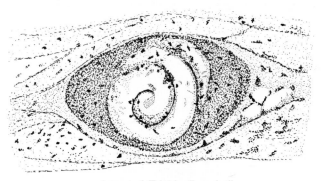

Larva of *Trichinella spiralis*

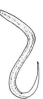

Larva of
Strongyloides stercoralis

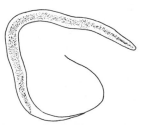

Larva of
Dracunculus medinensis

45μm

Fig. 7.2   Immature stages of Nematodes.

and increase in size to about 2 mm. They then break through into the alveoli, reaching there about 15 days after the original infection. From the alveoli the larvae crawl up the bronchi and trachea, then traverse the larynx and pharynx and are once more swallowed. The larvae pass down the oesophagus to the stomach and settle in the upper part of the small intestine. Here the final moult occurs, between the twenty-fifth and twenty-ninth day of infection. This migration through the lungs will take place in guinea pigs and rodents, as well as in the natural hosts — but in unnatural hosts the worms pass right through the intestine and are voided with the faeces. In the natural hosts, the larvae settle down in the upper part of the small intestine and become sexually mature in about 2 months. The length of life in the final host averages only 9–12 months.

Morphologically similar worms are found in pigs, but these worms are physiologically distinct from those found in man and are placed in a different species, *A. suum*. Man is only rarely infected with pig ascariasis. In some countries heavy infection with *A. lumbricoides* is associated with polluted water supplies, but more usually infection results from contamination of hands and food by eggs developing in soil in the vicinity of houses. Infections are most common where soil is polluted by faeces from young children and infants.

Medical aspects of ascariasis

Pathogenesis

Vast numbers of children harbour *A. lumbricoides*, and its harmful effects are often underestimated. During their 10 days' stay in the pulmonary capillaries and alveoli the migrating larvae may induce a transient pneumonitis with cough, expectoration, wheezing, fever and eosinophilia. This can be serious, sometimes being complicated by bacterial bronchopneumonia. Heavy *Ascaris* infections in children may cause colicky abdominal pains after food and anorexia. Nutritional deprivation results from the high metabolic demands of the worm. A heavy load of worms (perhaps up to 5 per cent of the child's weight) absorb a significant proportion of a marginal diet from the small intestine, and may further interfere with digestion by secretion of an antiprotease.

Mechanical obstruction of the intestine by a bolus of worms is a major cause of intestinal obstruction in children under the age of 5 years, and it is said to occur each year in 0.2 per cent of those infected. Obstruction may be preceded by excessive activity of the worms following the administration of tetrachlorethylene or a febrile illness.

The first indication of infection may be the vomiting of a roundworm, or passage of a worm in the stool during a febrile illness. Perforation of intestinal suture lines by *Ascaris* after surgical anastomosis may lead to peritonitis, and intestinal operations should be preceded by deworming where possible. Worms can migrate into and obstruct the appendix, common bile duct and pancreas causing appendicitis, obstructive jaundice and pancreatitis respectively. Bile duct migration can result in multiple liver abscesses, sometimes causing death.

Clinical findings

Most people with light infections are not seriously affected, but children with heavy infections suffer symptoms arising from the pathological effects described above. Heavily infected children are often malnourished and pot-bellied, and complain of abdominal pains.

Intestinal obstruction involves the small intestine, causing severe mid-abdominal pain, vomiting and absolute constipation. Bile duct obstruction causes jaundice, cholangitis and liver abscess formation with fever and pain in the liver area. Pneumonitis may be seasonal and occur in epidemics. Diagnosis of pulmonary ascariasis is difficult, but *Ascaris* larvae may be found in the sputum or gastric washings, and eosinophilia is present.

Treatment

Several anthelminthics are effective. Piperazine citrate in doses of 75 mg/kg daily for 2 days paralyses the worms, which are then swept out of the gut. Levamisole 5 mg/kg in one dose, pyrantel pamoate 10 mg/kg in one dose; and mebendazole 100 mg 2 times a day for 3 days are also effective. The advantage of the latter is that it is also effective in treating hookworm and *Trichuris* infections, which are often associated with ascariasis.

Intestinal obstruction, if diagnosed as due to ascariasis, is usually treated conservatively by administering piperazine citrate 60 mg/kg 12-hourly for 3–4 doses by a nasogastric tube; intestinal suction and intravenous fluids are also needed. If this fails, laparotomy and 'milking' the bolus past the ileocaecal valve is attempted, or enterostomy followed by removal of the worms. Diagnosis is aided by finding heavy egg excretion in the stools, and by small-volume contrast radiography of the intestine.

Bile duct obstruction due to *Ascaris* is difficult to diagnose definitively. If suspected, it is justifiable to observe the patient for 2 weeks before surgical exploration of the bile duct as the worm often retreats back into the bowel.

Toxocara canis

The dog ascarid *T. canis* and the morphologically similar cat ascarid *T. cati* are common throughout the world in domestic and wild canines and felines, although in some areas they are replaced by *Toxascaris leonina*. Man may become infected if he accidentally ingests the eggs of these worms, which are passed in the animals' faeces. Infection is commonest in children, probably because children are more likely than adults to ingest contaminated soil.

As man is an abnormal host, the larvae that hatch from the eggs develop only as far as the second, migratory stage. The larvae then move through the body as 'visceral larvae migrans' until they die, probably after some months. After penetrating the intestinal wall the larvae migrate to the liver; they may remain in the liver, or may migrate or be carried in the blood to the lungs and other parts of the body. When in the liver they may cause liver enlargement and fever and when in the lungs they may cause pulmonary signs and symptoms. Occasionally larvae may settle in the eye and cause blindness.

Medical aspects of toxocariasis

Pathogenesis and clinical picture

Visceral larva migrans is the term applied to the prolonged migration of nematode larvae in the deep tissues of man. It is usually the cat and dog ascarids involved in the cases to show characteristic symptoms. The condition is most frequently seen in young children, and the infections are associated with eosinophilic granulomata around larvae in various organs. Infected children may have irregular fever and muscular pains, and show loss of appetite. Pulmonary involvement is common, with cough and sometimes wheezing; hepatomegaly may be present, and marked eosinophilia is constant. The symptoms are usually mild but they may persist for months.

The most serious manifestation of toxocariasis is the formation of an eosinophilic granuloma in the retina of a child. This is visible by the opthalmoscope and has sometimes been mistaken for a glioblastoma, and the eye has been enucleated. The retinal lesion usually occurs in older children and is not associated with visceral symptoms. Diagnosis depends on clinical suspicion, the recognition of eosinophilia, and the results of serological tests using ELISA and immunofluorescence techniques.

Control

Children become infected by ingestion of eggs of *T. canis* or, less often, *T. cati* which have developed to the infective stage in the soil about two weeks after their passage in dogs' or cats' faeces. Prevention is difficult because of the crawling and eating habits of young children. Regular deworming of dogs and puppies is important in prevention.

Treatment

Thiabendazole 25 mg/kg 2 times a day for 7 days has proved effective in treatment. Eye lesions may need local treatment with photocoagulation.

Superfamily Oxyuroidea

These are mostly small or medium-sized worms in which there is an enlargement or 'bulb' at the posterior end of the oesophagus. The males have one or two copulatory spicules, and the tail of the female is usually slender and pointed.

Enterobius vermicularis

This is commonly called the pinworm or threadworm, and like *Ascaris* it is cosmopolitan in distribution. It is commoner in white than in black races, and commoner in cold and temperate climates then in warm climates. Unlike most human helminthic infections it is relatively rare in the tropics, perhaps because underclothes are worn less frequently in hot climates.

The adult worms live mainly in the caecum, appendix and lower ileum, and from these places the gravid females migrate to the rectum. The worms generally remain on the surface of the mucosa, but they may occasionally encyst in the submucosa. The cuticle, near the mouth in both sexes, is expanded laterally into alae. The mouth has three small lips. The male is about 4 mm in length and the female about 1 cm in length. The posterior extremity of the male is curved and sharply truncated, and bears a single hook-like spicule. The tail of the female is long, tapering, straight and pointed (Fig. 7.1).

Unlike all other nematodes parasitic in the intestine of man, *Enterobius* does not lay eggs in the intestine. As the uterus of the female fills with eggs, the worm migrates down to the anus. They creep out of the anus, or are passed with the faeces. When they come into contact with the air the worms begin to lay eggs, and a trail of these is left as the worm crawl across the skin. The worms usually die after egg-laying. The movement of the worms causes intense itching, and the worms are often crushed by the infected individual while scratching, thus releasing more eggs.

The average number of eggs in a single female has been estimated at about 11 000. The eggs regain access to the same person, or gain access to another person, in various ways, but probably they are most commonly transferred to the mouth on fingers that have scratched the perianal skin. Eggs on clothing or bedding may be transferred to the mouth via the fingers, or inhaled in dust. The infected households, the eggs may be found on clothing, bed linen, towels, soap, unholstery and furniture in every room.

When it is laid the egg (Fig. 7.2) contains a tadpole-like larva, which completes its development in 6–24 hours. When the egg is ingested, the shell is dissolved in the small intestine, and here the larva undergoes two further moults and develops to an adult without migrating from the intestine. The life-cycle from egg to adult takes 2–4 weeks.

It has been suggested that occasionally the moist environment causes the eggs to hatch on the skin in the perianal region, following which the larvae migrate up the bowel and develop there into adults — so called retrofection.

Medical aspects of *E. vermicularis* infection

Pathogenesis and clinical features

Enterobius inhabits the mucosa of the caecum, colon and lower ileum. It probably causes no serious pathology in the gut, although it is sometimes found in removed appendices and blamed for appendicitis in these cases.

The nocturnal migration of the female worm to lay eggs on the perianal skin is associated with local irritation — *pruritus ani*. Pruritus is in part due to local skin sensitization to eggs or worm products. A perianal eczematous reaction can result, and local bacterial skin infections may arise as a result of scratching. Insomnia due to *pruritus ani* causes lassitude and irritability. Some sufferers become obsessed with their infection, constantly inspecting their stools for worms and believing their infection is incurable. Indeed, it may recur at intervals for many years.

In females the worms sometimes migrate into the vagina, causing vaginal discharge and irritation. Rarely a granulomatous fallopian tube infection is attributed threadworms, and occasionally cystitis. Many individuals appear to have no symptoms despite threadworm infection.

Treatment

Because of persistence of viable *Enterobius* eggs in the environment for 2-3 weeks, reinfection is common after treatment; cure can be difficult. Eggs may persist in clothes, bed linen, dust and on door handles and toys. The infection is often present in several members of a family, some of whom may be asymptomatic.

Mebendazole 100 mg in one dose is convenient and effective. It is wise to repeat the treatment at one or two week intervals for 8-10 weeks, and simultaneously treat other members of the household. This makes reinfection less likely. Measures to avoid infection are advisable, including washing hands before food and after defaecation, keeping the nails short and clean, and bathing daily, preferably on rising. Pyrantel pamoate 10 mg/kg as one dose repeated weekly for 8-10 weeks is an alternative to mebendazole. Piperazine citrate is another drug formerly much used, but it requires 8 days' treatment at a dose of 65 mg/kg per day.

Clinical diagnosis

The problem is usually that of deciding the cause of the *pruritus ani*. Many cases of *pruritus ani* are not parasitic in origin, and may be associated with moniliasis, haemorrhoids, psychogenic problems or inadequate anal hygiene. *Taenia* and *Strongyloides* are other helminth parasites that may also cause pruritus.

Superfamily Trichuroidea

The members of this superfamily have bodies divided into two more or less distinct parts, the anterior one of which contains the oesophagus and the posterior one the remaining organs. The oesophagus is not muscular, and consists of a narrow capillary-like tube passing through a column of thin-walled cells. In some genera the anterior portion of the body is thin and hair-like and the posterior portion is thick. In all members of the superfamily the females possess only one ovary. The superfamily contains two genera (and two species) of considerable medical importance, *Trichuris trichiura* and *Trichinella spirallis*; and also one species of another genus, *Capillaria philippinensis*, which is less widespread but causes serious disease in parts of the Philippines and Thailand.

Trichuris trichiura

This worm, commonly known as the whipworm because of its shape, is cosmopolitan in distribution but is more common in warm moist regions. Trichurids that are morphologically very similar to those found in man can be found in practically all mammals, and occur plentifully in sheep and cattle. The adult worms are found in the caecum of their host, and may also occur in the ileum, appendix and colon.

The general shape of the worm is whip-like, with a hair-like anterior portion about three-fifths of the length of the worm and a much stouter posterior two-fifths (Fig. 7.1). The narrow anterior portion contains the oesophagus, and the worm bores into the wall of the intestine and settles with the whole of the anterior portion buried in the mucosa. The worm secretes a digestive fluid into the tissues around the mouth, and this converts the tissues into a liquid which the worm sucks up.

The male is about 4 cm in length and 2 mm wide in the thicker portion, and the posterior end is spirally coiled. The cloaca is terminal, and there is a single copulatory spicule.

The female is slightly larger, about 5 cm long, and the same width as the male. The vulva is situated near the junction of the two parts of the body.

The eggs develop in damp soil, and become infective after about 4 weeks, by which time they contain a fully developed larva. The eggs containing the infective larvae may remain viable for many months in suitable damp conditions. Man becomes infected by swallowing the embryonated egg, usually with contaminated food. When swallowed, the egg hatches to release the larva, which migrates to the caecum and develops into the adult worm.

Medical aspects of trichuriasis

Pathogenesis and clinical manifestations

The anterior ends of the worms are embedded in the mucosa of the colon, causing superficial inflammatory changes and minor haemorrhage. Each worm may cause the loss of 0.005 ml of blood daily; a load of 800 worms or more can eventually cause anaemia. Most infections are light, with loads of less than 100 worms. In heavy infections worms move down the large bowel from the caecum and can be seen in the rectum on proctoscopy. Heavy infections in children cause chronic diarrhoea, anaemia and rectal prolapse, and in Malaysia have been shown to be associated with malnutrition and increased liability to invasive amoebiasis.

Many infections are asymptomatic, but this very common helminth may have been underestimated as a pathogen. If the stool egg count is over 3000 eggs per gram, treatment is indicated.

Treatment

Mebendazole 100 mg 2 times a day for 3 days is the most effective treatment. Repeated courses may be needed.

Trichinella spiralis

This worm is cosmopolitan among pork-eating people. Essentially it is a parasite of rats, in which animals it produces an infection that is both enzootic and epizootic, but it has been recorded in a large number of animals. Different animals differ in their susceptibility; pigs and man are particularly susceptible.

The adult worms (Fig. 7.1) live in the duodenum and jejunum of their host. The male is about 1.5 mm long and 40 μm wide, so it is difficult to see with the naked eye and hence is rarely found. The posterior end is armed with a pair of small conical fleshy flaps shielding the terminal cloaca. The female is about twice the size of the male, 3 mm long and 60 μm wide. The vulva is situated about halfway along the oesophagus.

In both sexes the anterior portion of the body is filled by the oesophagus, but unlike in the whipworms there is no obvious difference in thickness between the two parts of the body.

T. spiralis differs from other nematodes of medical importance in that, while two hosts are necessary for the completion of the life cycle, each host contains both the adult and the larval stages. The adult worms are short-lived, and usually die about 3 months after the host has become infected, but they reach maturity within a few days of being ingested. After fertilization the females burrow into the wall of the small intestine. The fertilized eggs are retained in the uterus of the female worm until they hatch, and the larvae (not the eggs) are liberated by the worm about 5 days after infection of the host. These larvae are about 100 × 6 μm in size, and are carried either via the blood or via the lymph to the heart, and thence to all parts of the body. Only those which reach striated muscle survive, and the muscles most commonly infected are the very active ones such as those of the diaphragm, tongue, throat, eyes and thorax. Cardiac muscle is not usually affected. The larvae penetrate into the muscle and grow to a size of about 1 mm, this growth taking about 3 weeks. The fully grown larvae (now infective) coil up between the muscle fibres, and a lemon-shaped cyst forms around them (Fig. 7.2). The cysts usually measure not more than 500 × 200 μm, and each may contain several larvae. The larvae in the cyst may remain viable for as long as 30 years, but more frequently the cyst and larvae become calcified within a few months.

Man usually acquires the infection by eating insufficiently cooked pork or pork products. Infected pork may contain several thousands of infective larvae per gram, and a single adult female worm is estimated to produce about 1500 larvae after fertilization, so ingestion of a gram of such meat could produce at least a million encysted larvae. The pig becomes infected by eating infected rats, or more usually by eating infected flesh from other pigs fed to it in swill. In the intestine the gastric juices dissolve the cyst and liberate the larvae, which penetrate the epithelium of the intestine and mature within a few days.

Medical aspects of trichinosis

Pathogenesis

Adult worms develop from the infective larvae ingested in undercooked meat about five days earlier, and invade the jejunal mucosa. This produces an initial diarrhoeal illness lasting a few days. If the infection is recognized as trichinosis and treated at this stage, more serious consequences can be avoided. About a week later the viviparous female worm produces larvae which reach the blood stream via the intestinal lymphatics and the thoracic duct. Larval discharge may last 4–6 weeks or even longer. The larvae disseminate widely, but only those lodging in voluntary muscles survive and encyst. The diaphragm, intercostal muscles, extraocular muscles, masseters, pectoral girdle, gastrocnemius and tongue are particularly affected. Voluntary muscle fibres are invaded and degenerate, becoming surrounded by an inflammatory cellular reaction including eosinophils. Within a few weeks the now infective larva is surrounded by a fibrous capsule, and this calcifies in one or two years; these calcified areas are too small to be seen on routine X-rays. In other tissue such as the brain, heart and lungs the larvae degenerate and become surrounded by granulomata. These multiple granulomata cause encephalitis, myocarditis and pneumonitis.

The severity of the illness produced depends on the number of larvae disseminated. Most of those infected are asymptomatic or mildly ill, and not diagnosed. These people have fewer then 10 cysts per gram in biopsied, digested muscle. Seriously affected patients will have 50 or more cysts per gram of muscle. Immune processes develop which act on circulating larvae, inhibit reproduction of female worms, and possibly aid expulsion from the gut.

Clinical picture

A few days after eating undercooked pork, sausages, warthog or bear meat heavily infected with *Trichinella*, there is a diarrhoeal illness with abdominal pains lasting several days. One or two weeks later a febrile illness with severe muscular pains begins. This may last for 6 weeks. There is often difficulty and pain on respiration owing to involvement of the intercostal muscles and diaphragm, and the patient is prostrated. Oedematous swelling around the orbits and haemorrhage under the nails are common, and sometimes a cutaneous erythematous macular eruption is seen.

Serious complications include myocarditis with tachycardia, cardiac enlargement, cardiac failure and arrhythmias. Brain involvement causes encephalitic symptoms with mental confusion, headache, drowsiness and occasional focal signs such as hemiplegia. Pneumonitis with cough and expectoration results from pulmonary involvement. Occasional fatalities occur in heavily infected patients.

Clinical diagnosis

The initial diarrhoeal illness is difficult to differentiate from bacterial or viral gastroenteritis, except during a known outbreak, because larvae are not found in the stools. The early febrile illness needs differentiation from typhoid and poliomyelitis. Brain involvement mimics cerebral abscess or viral encephalitis, while myocarditis resembles rheumatic carditis.

Periorbital oedema, haemorrhages under the nails and eosinophilia are important diagnostic pointers that should lead to definitive laboratory diagnostic tests. The creatine phosphokinase and SGOT enzyme levels are raised.

Prevention

Trichinosis is a parasitic disease that could be prevented by proper cooking of food, and health education can play a part in prevention. Pig swill should be cooked before feeding to pigs, and rats should be excluded from slaughter houses. Cysts in meat cannot be detected by naked eye examination, and a special microscope called a trichinoscope has been used to detect cysts in tongue and other flesh. However, adequate inspection of meat is difficult.

Treatment

Thiabendazole in doses of 25 mg/kg 2 times a day for 5 days acts on the adults in the intestine, and to a lesser extent on the larvae. To be most successful it should be used before the larvae are disseminated, but this is rarely possible.

In the seriously ill patients, particularly those with myocarditis or encephalitis, prednisone in initial doses of 40–60 mg per day is given and gradually reduced after 5 days.

Capillaria

Capillaria hepatica is an infection of rodents and other animals in many parts of the world. Infections have occasionally been recorded in man. The adult worms live in the tissues of the host liver, and the eggs become trapped in the liver parenchyma. If infected liver is eaten by a carnivore, the eggs are freed when the liver tissue is digested and are then passed in the faeces of the carnivore. They develop in the soil to the infective embryonated stage, and susceptible animals (including man) are infected by ingesting the embryonated eggs in food or water. The infection in man can be fatal, with progressive liver damage and finally liver failure.

Another species, *C. philippinensis*, is a parasite of man in some parts of the Philippines and Thailand. The adult worms are small, the male being about 2.5 mm long and the female about 3.5 mm long, and they burrow into the mucous membrane of the small intestine, mainly in the jejunum. They initially cause signs of malabsorption and diarrhoea and some fatal cases have been recorded.

The eggs, which are passed in the faeces, are about 45 μm long. They are somewhat like the eggs of *Trichuris*, but the polar plugs do not protrude and the surface of the egg shell is pitted (Fig. 7.2). The eggs develop in the soil and become embryonated in about two weeks. The life-cycle is not known. Man is the only host found naturally infected, and infection apparently follows the ingestion of raw freshwater fish.

Medical aspects of intestinal capillariasis

Pathogenesis and clinical picture

Infection with *C. philippinensis* frequently causes serious illness. Invasion of the jejunal mucosa by large numbers of adult worms produces mucosal damage, with malabsorption and a protein-losing enteropathy.

The incubation period is 21–60 days. Initial symptoms include abdominal discomfort and borborygmi. Within 2–3 weeks, severe watery diarrhoea begins.

The clinical picture is a result of malabsorption and electrolyte depletion with hypokalaemia, hypocalcaemia and hypoalbuminaemia. Weakness, wasting, vomiting, oedema and hyporeflexia are other findings. Without treatment the mortality rate is about 10 per cent within 2–3 months.

Treatment

Mebendazole 100 mg 4 times a day for 20–30 days is administered. Thiabendazole has been used in doses of 25 mg/kg daily in 2 doses for 1 month; it is more toxic than mebendazole.

Supportive therapy to correct electrolyte depletion and malnutrition is also needed.

Superfamily Ancylostomatoidea

The worms of this superfamily have one easily recognizable characteristic which is almost constant and is peculiar to them, namely a 'bursa' surrounding the cloaca of the male. The bursa is an umbrella-like expansion of the cuticle at the end of the body which is supported by fleshy rays comparable with the ribs of an umbrella. Usually the bursa consists of three lobes, two lateral and one dorsal, and it may or may not be split ventrally. It varies in size, and in some of the lung worms (Metastrongylidae) it is vestigeal or even absent. The oesophagus is muscular and is club-shaped or cylindrical; and the mouth has no lips. The mouth may be a simple opening or there may be a distinct buccal cavity. The eggs have thin transparent colourless shells (Fig. 7.2). When laid they contain either a divided ovum (a morula) or a larva. The egg hatches outside the body to produce a free-living larva that enters the new host either by burrowing through the skin, by being ingested with water or vegetation, or (in some of the lung worms) via an intermediate host. The superfamily contains two species that are parasitic in man, namely *Ancylostoma duodenale* and *Necator americanus*, both of which possess a large buccal capsule lined with chitin which is developed into cutting organs. In *Ancylostoma* these are tooth-like, in *Necator* they are plate-like. The anterior end of the worms is curled into a hook — hence the name hookworm.

Hookworms exist where local conditions are favourable in most tropical and subtropical parts of the world, and they may be endemic wherever freezing temperatures do not last long and where standards of hygiene are low. In temperate climate they may occur in special situations such as mines.

Ancylostoma duodenale

This is primarily a northern species and predominates in southern Europe, North Africa, Western Asia, northern Chia and Japan, but it has been carried by man to all parts of the world. It is larger and coarser than *Necator*, the males being about 9 mm long and the females 12 mm long (Fig. 7.1). The mature worms are cylindrical, rigid and creamy-white, although freshly expelled specimens have a dirty rust colour due to ingested blood. The anterior end of the worms is slightly curved dorsally. The cuticle is finely striated transversely. The mouth opens into a large buccal cavity lined with chitin. The mouth is oval (the transverse axis being the longer) and two teeth are visible on either side of the ventral margin. There is another pair of teeth deep inside the buccal cavity. On the ventral side is also a pair of glands which open between the teeth and probably secrete an anticoagulant or histolytic substance.

The oesophagus arises at the base of the buccal cavity. It is club-shaped, and measures about one-sixth of the length of the worm. The male is about 9 mm long and 500 μm wide. The posterior end of the body is expanded to form the copulatory bursa. The cloaca is terminal, and there are two protrusible copulatory spicules. The female is about 12 mm long and 600 μm wide. The anus is subterminal, and at the posterior end of the body is a caudal spine. The vulva is at the junction of the middle and posterior third of the body.

A. duodenale is primarily a human parasite, but on rare occasions it has been found in pigs, and experimentally it can sometimes be reared in cats, dogs and monkeys. Another species, *A. ceylanicum*, is an occasional human parasite in South East Asia and India. *A. brasiliense*, normally a parasite of cats and dogs in Africa and Central and South America, is a cause of 'creeping eruption'.

Necator americanus

This is primarily a tropical worm. It is now the predominant species in all parts of the world except those mentioned above as the localities for *A. duodenale*. It is called the 'American hookworm' because it was first discovered in America, but it is probably African in origin. It is smaller and more slender than *Ancylostoma*, the females averaging about 11 mm in length and the males about 8 mm (Fig. 7.1). The head in both sexes is finer than that of *Ancylostoma*, and is bent more sharply dorsally; this latter characteristic is probably the simplest way to differentiate the species. The vulva of the female is situated near the middle of the body (further forward than that of *Ancylostoma*) and there is no caudal spine. The bursa in the male is longer and narrower than that of *Ancylostoma*, and is distinguished by the split dorsal ray and the approximation of two of the lateral rays. In *Ancylostoma* the dorsal ray is not divided, and the three lateral rays are spread nearly equally.

The armature of the buccal cavity differs from that of *Ancylostoma* in that the ventral cutting organs consist of two semilunar plates, not teeth, and that in addition to the two subventral teeth (which are also possessed by *Ancylostoma*) there are two subdorsal teeth in *Necator*.

The adult hookworms of both genera live in the upper part of the small intestine of man, particularly in the jejunum and less often in the duodenum. The worms draw a piece of the mucous membrane into their buccal capsule, and nourish themselves on blood and tissue juices they suck.

Estimates show that the female *Ancylostoma* produces about 15 000 eggs per day, and *Necator* about half that number. At any one time, however, the uterus of the worm contains about 5 per cent of that number. The eggs are passed in the faeces and do not develop further until exposed to the air in warm and damp conditions.

After about 24 hours the first-stage larva hatches, and in the tropics the speed of development is increased by dung beetles which stir up and aerate the faeces. When hatched, the larva has an oesophagus about half the length of the intestinal tract, has a rounded anterior end and a pointed tail, and is about 250 μm in length. After about 3 days the larva moults to produce the second-stage larva, which is similar to the first-stage but about 500 μm long. After another week a second moult occurs to produce the infective third-stage larva, which is filariform (i.e. it has a tubular oesophagus and not one with a bulb) and about 600 μm long. The third-stage larva retains the cast cuticle of the previous stage as a sheath, and it is rapidly killed by freezing, desiccation, direct sunlight and certain chemicals. The sheath remains until the larva penetrates the host skin, when it is cast off. The larvae burrow until they enter a lymp- or blood-vessel, and are finally carried via the heart to the lungs, where they are filtered out in the capillaries and burrow through into the air spaces of the lungs. They then pass up the trachea, over the epiglottis, down the oesophagus and through the stomach to the duodenum. Only those larvae that reach the lungs complete their development. The third moult takes place a few days later in the duodenum or small intestine, and the fourth-stage larva possesses a temporary buccal capsule with the typical adult armature. This larva grows and feeds until it reaches a length of about 4 mm, when the fourth moult occurs. The worm now possesses a fully developed buccal capsule, and the reproductive organs become mature in about a week (5 weeks or so after penetration). In man the eggs first appear in the faeces about 6 weeks after penetration, and the adult worm may live for 5 years or more.

Hookworm larvae normally live in the upper centimetre or so of soil, and commonly climb up to the highest points to which a film of moisture extends — on soil particles, dead vegetation etc. On these they extend their bodies into the air and await a chance to apply themselves to animal skin. When exposed to a hot sun or superficial drying of soil, they retreat into crevices in the upper layer of soil. They do not migrate laterally to any great extent, but they are dispersed by insects, rain etc. In loose-textured soil they can migrate vertically by as much as a metre, but from trenches or pits they do not climb the walls but stop at the tips of any projecting particles.

The larvae are strongly attracted by moderate heat, and are stimulated to activity by contact with solid objects; and it is the combination of these reactions that causes them to burrow into the skin of animals. Infection normally takes place by the larvae penetrating the skin, usually of bare feet. But less frequently infection results from the ingestion of water or food harbouring infective larvae.

Medical aspects of hookworm infection

Pathogenesis

The serious effects of heavy hookworm infection are caused by chronic haemorrhage from the duodenal and jejunal mucosa. Hookworms ingest blood, and when they move to a new attachment site (probably several times daily) the haemorrhage continues from the old site because of an anticoagulant secreted by the worm. One *Ancylostoma* uses about 0.15 ml of blood per day while a *necator* uses 0.05 ml. The worms excrete waste products and perhaps 50 per cent of the iron in the lost blood is reabsorbed. If the patient's iron intake is outstripped by blood loss, depletion of the body's iron stores results and an iron deficiency anaemia follows. Loss of plasma protein causes hypoalbuminaemia in those on a poor diet. The constant loss of as little as 10 ml of blood a day can eventually cause severe anaemia, contribute to malnutrition, and stunt the mental and physical development of a child. The magnitude of the effects of hookworm infection depends on the number of worms present, the species of worm, the iron reserves of the host, the duration of infection and the dietary intake of iron. It has been estimated that hookworms cause the loss of 7 million litres of blood daily from 700 million people.

Sometimes hookworms cause epigastric pain, as can other worms attached to the small intestinal mucosa. Barium meals may show irregularity of the duodenal outline described as duodenitis, but pathologically there is only superficial mucosal damage. The pain can closely resemble that due to peptic ulcer.

Itchy papular eruptions lasting a few days appear at the site of larval invasion — usually on the feet between the toes. This eruption is known as ground itch, it is by no means always found, and it is of little clinical significance unless there is secondary bacterial infection. During early larval migration through the lungs, larval pneumonitis with cough, expectoration and wheezing may occur, but it is less common and less severe than in ascariasis. Malabsorption is now considered extremely uncommon in hookworm disease.

Immunity in hookworm infection is not well understood. The adult lumenal worm with poorly antigenic surface cuticle living several years in the gut is probably not destroyed by immune processes. There may be immune destruction of tissue-traversing larvae, limiting super infection. Greatly differing worm loads of individuals apparently equally exposed to infection, and frequent failure of heavy recolonization of the gut after treatment, suggest that some immune process is at work.

Clinical features

Only a small proportion of people with hookworm infection show signs of illness with hookworm disease. The symptoms and signs are of a slowly progressing anaemia with lassitude, diminished capacity for physical and mental work, headache, palpitations and pallor of mucous membranes. Eventually oedema and cardiac failure appear, often not apparent until the haemoglobin falls below 3–5 g/dl. Hypoalbuminaemia contributes to peripheral oedema. The cardiovascular system adapts remarkably well to a slowly developing anaemia by tachycardia and increased stroke volume; this causes palpitations, particularly on exercise, when the haemoglobin falls below 7 g/dl. Initially cardiac failure is hyperkinetic in type, with vasodilation, a large pulse pressure and a warm periphery. Eventually a low output state supervenes. Syncope in the upright position and mental confusion are grave signs of cerebral anoxia and impending collapse. Koilonychia is occasionally present.

Epigastric pain may mimic peptic ulceration. Caution is necessary in attributing abdominal pain to intestinal worms. Many people have hookworm infection without pain. It is necessary to treat the patient, ensure that the worm load has been markedly lessened, and confirm that the pain has disappeared — if not, further investigation is needed. Pica and perverted appetite, particularly for earth or clay, has been attributed to hookworm. Pica leads to polyparasitism and rarely intestinal obstruction. Ground itch and pneumonitis are relatively uncommon and usually minor problems. There is some controversy about susceptibility to other infections in hookworm anaemia. Malaria and amoebiasis appear to be suppressed during iron deficiency and recur with renewed virulence during replenishment of iron stores following hookworm treatment.

Incapacity for physical work, stunting of physical development, aggravation of malnutrition and increased risk in pregnancy are serious community problems in areas of widespead hookworm infection.

Clinical diagnosis

Hypochromic anaemia is the usual presentation. It is necessary to link this with hookworm infection and to consider other possible causes such as piles, bleeding peptic ulcer, menorrhagia etc. Usually a faecal egg count of at least 2000 eggs per gram of faeces is necessary to imply causation of hypochromic anaemia by hookworms. The stools are positive for occult blood, but macroscopic blood in the stools or melaena are rarely seen. Blood films show hypochromia and microcytosis; the mean corpuscular haemoglobin concentration is below 30 per cent; the serum iron is low, and stainable iron is absent from the marrow. Eosinophilia may be present, particularly in the early stages of primary infection. Serum albumin is often low.

Management

The first priority is treatment of the anaemia. Moderate anaemia is treated with oral iron compounds, which are well tolerated by most indigenous people. Ferrous sulphate 300 mg is administered once on the first day, twice the second day, and three times daily thereafter. It is better tolerated and reasonably well absorbed if given after a light meal. It is necessary to continue treatment for several months to restore the haemoglobin to normal and replenish the iron stores. Ferrous gluconate is a more expensive alternative. Intravenous iron dextran by total dose infusion is a more toxic and expensive treatment, and is usually unnecessary. It can be justified if there are serious compliancy, intolerance or absorption problems.

Life-threatening anaemia with severe cardiac failure and syncope is treated by blood transfusion. Blood transfusion in such patients is hazardous because of the danger of precipitating fatal pulmonary oedema. A slow transfusion of 500 ml of packed red cell suspension is administered slowly over 8 hours; 40 mg of frusemide is given intravenously at the start of the transfusion. The patient is monitored for dyspnoea, cough, increasing jugular venous pressure and basal crepitations. The appearance of these signs of pulmonary congestion necessitates cessation of infusion, oxygen and further intravenous diuretics. If necessary, slow transfusion can be repeated after 24–48 hours. Exchange transfusion is now rarely necessary. Cardiac failure is treated with diuretics in moderate dosage; digoxin is of dubious benefit.

Specific treatment is given to remove the worms. Pyrantel pamoate 10 mg/kg in one dose (maximum 1 gm); mebendazole 100 mg 2 times a day for 3 days; or bitosconate 100 mg (not for children) can all be used. Pyrantel is also effective against *Ascaris*, and mebendazole against *Ascaris* and *Trichuris*. Intestinal polyparasitism is common in hookworm sufferers. Tetrachlorethylene is used in doses of 5 ml for adults and 0.12 ml/kg for children; but if ascariasis is present it must be treated first as tetrachlorethylene may precipitate intestinal obstruction by *Ascaris*. Many would advise treating severe anaemia for 2 weeks before giving anthelminthics. It is probably not justifiable to treat light hookworm infections, with scanty egg excretion, in an adult living in an endemic area.

There should be follow-up as necessary to ensure that egg excretion has ceased or reached low levels in the stools, and that the haemoglobin is increasing satisfactorily.

Cutaneous larva migrans

The two most common and important human hookworms, already described, are *Ancylostoma duodenale* and *Necator americanus*. However, infective filariform larvae of certain 'foreign' species of hookworms, in particular the dog hookworm *A. braziliense*, may penetrate into the skin of man but are unable to make their way below the stratum germinativum, and so are unable to reach blood or lymph vessels. They therefore wander aimlessly just under the skin surface, moving a few centimetres a day, sometimes for several months, causing tortuous itchy channels in the skin. This condition is known as cutaneous larva migrans or creeping eruption. The advancing end of the track is usually erythematous, painful and swollen, and there is often severe pruritus of the area. The severity of the reaction depends on the previous sensitization and the allergic responses of the individual. A similar effect is produced by larvae of the European dog hookworm, *Uncinaria stenocephala*, but in this case the eruption usually lasts only a few weeks. In highly sensitized individuals larvae of *A. caninum* may cause severe skin reactions, but they only rarely cause a typical creeping eruption.

Pathogenesis and clinical features

The migrating larvae produce erythematous papules and sinuous tracks, usually on the feet, legs or buttocks. Symptoms may continue for weeks or months. Scratching in response to the itch causes secondary bacterial infection. Occasionally there are transient pulmonary infiltrations with eosinophilia (Loeffler's syndrome).

Treatment

A 10 per cent suspension of thiabendazole in an ointment base, applied locally once daily for a few days, usually cures. Ten per cent metrifonate in an ointment base also works. If these fail, oral thiabendazole 25 mg/kg 2 times a day for 3 days should be given.

Other helminths moving under the skin may be seen, and may cause cutaneous larva margins, including *Strongyloides stercoralis* and *Gnathostoma spinigera*. The larva of *Gasterophilus* (the horse bot fly) will also cause a larva migrans — it is treated by removal with a needle.

Superfamily Gnathostomatoidea

Another form of visceral larva migrans may be caused by the larvae of *Gnasthostoma spinigerum*. This worm was first recorded in gastric tumours in a tiger, and has since been found in various cats (both wild and domestic) and in dogs in many parts of the world. Human infections have been recorded in Thailand, India, Malaysia, China, Japan and various Pacific Islands, but Thailand is the country where it is commonest in both the human and the reservoir hosts.

In their normal hosts the adult worms live in tunnels or tumours in the stomach wall. The worms are stout and reddish-coloured, with a globular swelling at the anterior end separated from the rest of the body by a constriction. This swelling is armed with 4–8 rows of sharp recurved hooks.

The eggs are passed in faeces and hatch to release the first first-stage larva. This larva is swallowed by a water-flea. *Cyclops*, within which it moults to a second-stage larva. When the *Cyclops* is eaten by a frog, fish or snake, the third-stage larva develops — and finally cats and dogs become infected by eating these second intermediate hosts.

Man may infect himself with the third-stage larvae by eating fish containing them, and if he does this the larvae may wander in the skin to produce local symptoms. The larvae in man do not become fully mature gnathostomes; only immature worms have been found in man, and these have been found in the peripheral tissues, usually subcutaneous. The worms in the skin may cause development of abscess pockets or of nodules with abscessed centres, or there may be a typical creeping eruption. The lesions may develop on any of the peripheral areas of the body, and are occasionally serious when the brain is involved.

It seems probable that man, like the normal hosts, acquires the infection by eating infected tissues of the second intermediate hosts. If this is the case, the larva must then migrate from the digestive tract to the superficial tissues. However, the possibility of infection through the skin has not been excluded.

Medical aspects of gnathostomiasis

Clinical manifestations

The most common clinical manifestations are the appearance of transient sub-cutaneous swellings, lasting a few days, in various parts of the body including the orbit. These swellings may itch but they are not acutely painful. Eosinophilia is common.

More serious symptoms occur if the worm migrates in deeper tissues, when it may cause severe abdominal pain, pneumothorax and haemoptysis. Rarely the central nervous system is invaded, and eosinophilic meningoencephalitis and bleeding into the cerebrospinal fluid may then result. This condition is often fatal.

Treatment

No effective curative drug therapy is known. Surgical excision of subcutaneous worms and destruction of these worms *in situ* by ultrasonic therapy have been used. Antihistamines and steroids provide some systematic relief. As usual, prevention is better than cure; and this entails the proper cooking of freshwater fish and chicken, and also of snakes and frogs if these animals are to be eaten.

Superfamily Rhabdiasoidea

This superfamily includes a number of minute worms that are either completely free-living or else in a state of adapting themselves to a parasitic way of life and leading an existence with alternating parasitic and free-living periods. The superfamily contains one genus of medical importance, *Strongyloides*. *Strongyloides* has various species which parasitize domestic and wild animals; and one species, *S. stercoralis*, is a widespread and fairly common parasite of man. It occurs chiefly in the wet tropics, in both the Old World and the New World, but it is occasionally recorded in temperate climates. Another species, *S. fuelleborni*, has been recorded occasionally infecting man, particularly in Africa; and a *fuelleborni*-like species is often found in infants in parts of Papua New Guinea.

Strongyloides stercoralis

As with all parasitic members of the superfamily, *S. stercoralis* has parasitic and free-living generations. The two developmental cycles overlap, and they do not necessarily succeed each other in any regular order. Probably the larvae that are passed in the faeces of the infected individual always develop in the soil into free-living males and females, but the larvae produced by these females may develop either into another free-living generation or into a parasitic generation. The sequence appears to be dependent mainly on the environmental conditions to which the larvae are exposed in the soil.

The adult parasitic females are slender, colourless worms, 2–2.5 mm in length and about 50 μm in breadth (Fig. 7.1). They are extremely difficult to detect either in biopsy material or in faeces. The 'parasitic male', which is morphologically similar to the free-living male, has been described from specimens that have been recovered from the gut of animals following experimental infections — but it has not been found in infections in man. Various authorities give different opinions regarding the presence or absence of adult males in the parasitic life-cycle, and whether the parasitic female is parthenogenetic.

The parasitic females burrow into the mucous membrane of the gut, chiefly in the small intestine, but they may invade any part of the gut from the duodenum to the rectum, or even lie free in the crypts between the villi. In these situations they lay their eggs, strung out in a chain by a thin, transparent, sheath-like membrane. The egg output is relatively small, and probably averages not more than 50 per day per worm.

Each egg, when passed, measures about 50 × 30 μm, and contains a fully developed larva inside a thick, clear shell. The larva hatches almost immediately, so that usually only larvae appear in the stool, although under conditions of intestinal hurry an occasional egg containing a larva may make its appearance. Normally the larvae hatching from the eggs make their way into the lumen of the gut and are voided with the faeces (Fig. 7.2).

The further development of the rhabditiform larvae may now follow one of two different lines, either direct or indirect. In the indirect case one or more free-living generations intervene before the parasite re-enters a human host.

The direct parasitic cycle proceeds as follows. The rhabditiform larvae in the soil or in the stool (*Strongyloides* larvae, unlike hookworm larvae, develop in faeces) grow, and after three or four days have moulted twice to become infective filariform larvae, which measure 0.5–0.6 mm in length and have a long simple tubular oesophagus. They closely resemble the infective filariform hook-worm larvae, but can be distinguished by the longer oesophagus (half the body length in *Strongyloides* compared with quarter the body length in hookworms), by the presence of a notch at the tip of the tail, and by the absence of the sheath. These infective larvae behave very similarly to hookworm larvae, inhabiting the upper inch of damp soil, and they can survive several weeks awaiting an opportunity to enter the final host. They are, however, more delicate than hookworm larvae, and can only survive for several weeks, compared with several months for hookworm larvae. They are much less resistant to desic-cation, excessive humidity and marked changes in temperature than are hookworm larvae. This inability to withstand low temperatures probably explains the comparative absence of *Strongyloides* from temperate and sub-tropical climates, while the sensitivity to desiccation accounts for its greater abundance in the wet tropics.

After the third-stage larva penetrates the skin of man, the subsequent life-cycle somewhat resembles those of *Ascaris* and the hookworms. When through the skin, the larvae enter the blood stream and are carried to, among other places, the lungs. In the lungs the developing larvae enter the alveoli, the bron-chioles and the bronchi. They then migrate up the trachea and down the oeso-phagus before undergoing the final two moults prior to reaching maturity in the alimentary canal. After being fertilized, the females burrow into the intestinal mucosa and commence the egg-laying cycle. The complete cycle of devel-opment, from penetration of the skin to the appearance of larvae in the faeces, occupies 2–3 weeks.

If the third-stage larvae do not penetrate the skin of man to commence the direct parasitic cycle, they develop into one or more generations of free-living, non-parasitic worms before resuming the parasitic habit. These free-living males and females mate, and the females subsequently lay eggs from which hatch rhabditiform larvae. These larvae either repeat the free-living cycle, or else develop to form filariform larvae that are indistinguishable from those produced by the parasitic generations of adults, and which are capable of piercing the skin of man and re-establising the parasitic cycle.

It is said that a person apparently unexposed to reinfection from outside may harbour an increasing population of *Strongyloides*. This is explainable by auto-infection. In such cases it is believed that newly hatched larvae in the gut may remain in the lumen of the gut, develop into filariform larvae, and burrow through the mucosa and into the blood vessels. They then develop normally, and reappear in the gut as adults. It has also beeen suggested that the rhab-ditiform larvae on the soiled skin of the perianal region may develop there into filariform larvae and then penetrate the skin, but this seems less likely. In any case, autoinfection appears to be uncommon.

Medical aspects of *S. stercoralis* infection (strongyloidiasis)

Pathogenesis and clinical effects

Infection with *S. stercoralis* is usually asymptomatic in indigenous people in the tropics, but it is more commonly symptomatic in expatriates. In heavy infec-tions, and in people with immune deficiency, strongyloidiasis can be serious and even fatal.

Itchy skin with erythematous tracks has been seen at the larval invasion site; transient pneumonitis with cough and expectoration may occur a few days after the infection as in hookworm larval migration.

Normally adult females inhabit the mucosa of the upper jejunum, but in heavy infections the whole small bowel, colon, biliary and pancreatic ducts may be colonized. Mucosal invasion causes inflammation with local macrophage and eosinophil accumulation, and may result in epigastric pain similar to that of peptic ulceration and diarrhoea. In heavy infections malabsorption may occur. Rarely ileus and intestinal obstruction follow small intestinal stasis, which may be induced by drugs such as diphenoxylate or even as a result of constipation.

Hyperinfection, with widespread larval dissemination in the tissues, is a serious complication in people harbouring *Strongyloides* whose immunity is depressed by corticosteroids, immunosuppressives or by serious malnutrition in childhood. The larvae and adults proliferate unchecked in the bowel, penetrate the intestinal wall, and spread to invade the peritoneum, liver, lungs, meninges and brain. This invasion is associated with Gram-negative septicaemia due to larval-borne intestinal bacteria. It is a grave and often lethal condition.

Autoinvasion of the bowel wall or perineum is followed by subcutaneous larval migration, the worms moving at a comparatively rapid rate — hence the term 'larva currens'. The itchy, erythematous, migrating larval tracks are found on the perineum, buttocks or trunk. Larva currens is a cause of pruritus ani. Because of repeated autoinfection, strongyloidiasis may persist for 40 years after the initial infection.

Various clinical results of strongyloidiasis are summarized in Table 7.1.

Table 7.1 Effects of infection with *Strongyloides stercoralis*

Type of stage of infection	Pathogenesis	Clinical effects
Early larval invasion	Larval skin penetration; pulmonary migration	Local itchy rash; transient pneumonitis (rarely diagnosed)
Light established infection	Autoinfection and larval wandering Invasion of jejunal mucosa.	Subcutaneous larva migrans, itchy erythematous tracks. Usually none
Heavy infection	Invasion of intestinal mucosa; marked local inflammatory changes	Epigastric pain, diarrhoea, malabsorption; rarely — ileus
Hyperinfection in immune-deficient host (steroids, immunosuppressives, malnutrition)	Massive larval production in the gut, penetration of intestinal wall, spread through body Gram-negative septicaemia	Peritonitis, pneumonitis, meningitis, encephalitis Septicaemic shock

Clinical diagnosis

Strongyloidiasis should be considered in people who have resided in warm climates and who show chronic digestive upsets, malabsorption or recurrent itchy linear skin rashes. Eosinophilia is usually present in those with symptomatic infections, but it is absent in the hyperinfection syndrome. The hyperinfection presents as a grave septicaemic illness with abdominal symptoms in the immunocompromized host. It is often unrecognized until post mortem examination. People who are at risk of *Strongyloides* infection must have their stools examined, and if necessary be treated for the infection, before the administration of steroids or immunosuppressives.

Treatment

Thiabendazole 25 mg/kg is given 12-hourly for 3 days. This drug may cause anorexia, nausea, vomiting, headache and drowsiness. Mebendazole 100 mg 3 times a day for 7 days has also been used. Subjects with symptoms due to strongyloidiasis, those who may need immunosuppressive or steroid treatment, and those who are permanently leaving an endemic area should be treated. The hyperinfection syndrome necessitates treatment with broad-spectrum bactericidal antibiotics, metronidazole, longer course of thiabendazole and intensive care.

Strongyloides fuelleborni

S. fuelleborni is a common parasite of Old World monkeys and apes which has sometimes been reported as an infection of man in parts of Africa. The adult female *S. fuelleborni* produces eggs, not larvae as does *S. stercoralis*, and these eggs appear in the faeces of an infected individual. The eggs in newly passed faeces are generally similar to those of the common hookworms, but they are smaller and measure about 50 × 35 μm. In addition, a *fuelleborni*-like parasite is endemic in some areas of Papua New Guinea.

The life-cycle and epidemiology of these two parasites are not fully known. Larvae of *S. fuelleborni* can be transmitted to human infants in the milk from nursing mothers, and it has been suggested that the *S. fuelleborni*-like parasite in Papua New Guinea is also transmitted through mothers' milk.

Medical aspects of S. fuelleborni-like parasite infection

Pathogenesis and clinical effects

Massive infection may occur in infants during the perinatal period. The infection may be heavy at the age of one month and increase up to the age of four months, after which it declines. The pathological changes are probably secondary to malabsorption, protein-losing enteropathy, and autoinfection with secondary bacterial infection. Clinical features include severe abdominal distension, mild diarrhoea, respiratory distress and, terminally, peripheral oedema. Without treatment many affected children die.

Laboratory findings include hypoproteinaemia with gross hypoalbumin-aemia, eosinophilia and anaemia.

Treatment

Thiabendazole 25 mg/kg 2 times a day for 3 days is often life-saving. Infusion of plasma, or of albumin and broad-spectrum antibiotics, is also indicted.

Superfamily Metastrongyloidea

Angiostrongylus cantonensis

A. cantonensis is a small worm, about 20 mm in length, which is a parasite of rodents in large areas of the tropics. Human infections with *Angiostrongylus* have been reported from Taiwan, Thailand, and the South Pacific, Indonesia, Vietnam, Malaysia, the Philippines, Papua New Guinea, Australia and other localities.

In rodent infections the adult worms live in the pulmonary blood vessels. The eggs are laid in the lung capillaries where they hatch, and the larvae migrate up the trachea and are passed out with the faeces. The larvae then penetrate into, or are ingested by, various land snails, and in these they develop into infective, third-stage larvae. If the snail is eaten by the rodent, the larvae migrate to the brain and develop to young adults; and finally they migrate to the pulmonary arteries where the females begin to lay eggs.

Hundreds of cases of human infection have been reported, but it is not known in all cases how the infection was obtained. The majority of infections are associated with eating raw or undercooked snails, especially the giant African snail *Achatina fulica*. However, many other species of snails and slugs are natural hosts of the infective larvae, and could be sources of human infections.

Angiostrongylus costaricensis

This is another parasite of rodents, found mainly in Central and South America, although naturally infected cotton rats have been recorded in the USA. The female worm is about 30 mm long and the male about 20 mm long, and they normally live in the mesenteric arteries of their host. The eggs are passed into the blood stream and hatch in the wall of the intestine to produce larvae which are then passed in the rodent's faeces. The larvae are ingested by slugs and develop into infective third-stage larvae. The rodents become infected by eating slugs containing the larvae.

Human infections have been recorded mainly in children, and have been reported in small numbers from several countries from Mexico to Brazil. The infections is best known in Costa Rica, where scores of cases are reported each year. In the areas where human infection has been recorded, raw slugs are not considered to be edible. If therefore seems probable that human infection follows the accidental ingestion of slugs (or of *Angiostrongylus* larvae that have emerged from slugs) with unwashed raw fruit or vegetables.

Medical aspects of angiostrongyliasis

Pathogenesis

Pathological changes in the brain and meninges result from eosinophilic granulomatous reactions to damaged and dead third-stage larvae. Migration of the larvae produces tunnels and cavities in the brain. Inflammatory response in the meninges results in a cellular exudate in the cerebrospinal fluid of 100–2000 cells per cubic millimetre, of which 20–75 per cent are eosinophils. Occasionally the larvae reach the eye and cause ocular damage. Infection does not induce immunity, and second attacks may occur.

Clinical features

Many cases are probably mild and transient; and the mortality rate is low, usually being under 1 per cent. The incubation period is 1–4 weeks and on average is about 2 weeks. Headache is often severe, bitemporal or occipital in site, and associated with nausea, vomiting and neck stiffness. Paraesthesiae are common and may persist for years. Low fever may be present, but it is often absent. In a few cases there is paresis of the seventh or sixth cranial nerves. Cauda equina lesions and myositis may occur. Eye lesions may cause retinal detachment and visual loss.

Diagnosis

The diagnosis must be considered in endemic areas in those with persistent headache. Examination of the cerebrospinal fluid shows an eosinophilic pleocytosis — which may also be caused by cerebral cysticercosis, cerebral paragonimiasis, coccidioidal meningitis and intrathecal injection of foreign proteins. There is often an eosinophilia in the blood. Rarely, larvae have been seen in the eye.

Treatment

Treatment is supportive and symptomatic. Analgesics are needed, and repeated drainage of 10 ml of cerebrospinal fluid is said to relieve headache. Assisted ventilation is required if respiration is paralysed. The value of corticosteroids is uncertain, and thiabendazole is considered possibly dangerous. Prevention of infection depends on health education, avoiding consumption of raw molluscs and paratenic hosts, and washing green vegetables free of slugs before consumption.

Abdominal angiostrongyliasis

Pathogenesis

The adult *A. costaricensis* localize in the ileocaecal region and lay eggs which do not hatch. Eosinophilic granulomas form in the area, with infiltration of the small intestine, caecum, appendix, ascending colon, and occasionally the liver. Worms may be found in mesenteric arteries causing arteritis and infarcts.

Clinical features and treatment

The disease usually occurs in children and presents with acute abdominal pain with prolonged fever, a mass in the right iliac fossa, and vomiting. There is a leucocytosis with 10 000–50 000 white blood cells per cubic millimetre, 10–80 per cent of which are eosinophils. Barium meal of the small intestine shows filling defects, irritability, and spasm of the small intestine.

There is no specific chemotherapy, and surgery may be needed.

Superfamily Filarioidea

The Filarioidea, commonly known as the filarias or the filarial worms, are long, slender, delicate, usually thread-like worms. The mouth is usually small and simple, without lips, and there is usually neither a buccal cavity nor a pharynx. The oesophagus is cylindrical, the anterior portion being muscular and the posterior portion glandular. In the females the vulva is situated near the anterior end of the body. The males are small, with coiled tails that may or may not bear alae but always bear papillae. The adult worms live in the tissues of the definitive host. The females usually give birth to fully developed larvae, known as microfilariae, which swarm in the blood or skin, and develop in bloodsucking insects.

Worms that parasitize man are usually 2–10 cm in length, though the female of one species, *Onchocerca volvulus*, is considerably longer. The adults live in the serous cavities, circulatory system, lymphatic system and connective tissue, but the species parasitizing man occur only in the last two sites. All members of the superfamily require an intermediate arthropod host, in which the microfilariae undergo further development before they become infective to the vertebrate host.

The Filaroidea have a world-wide distribution, and in Great Britain, for example, a considerable number of species of birds and mammals are hosts of various species of filariae. Those that parasitize man, however, are confined to the tropics. More than 20 species have been recorded from man, but only seven are sufficiently common to be of medical importance. These species are:

1. *Wuchereria bancrofti*
2. *Brugia malayi*
3. *Loa loa*
4. *Mansonella perstans*
5. *M. ozzardi*
6. *M. streptocerca*
7. *Onchocerca volvulus*

The adults of these seven species can be distinguished by differences in their morphology. However, since the adult worms are obtained only at autopsy or during surgical operations, diagnosis is usually based on an examination of the microfilariae found in the blood or skin. Recognition of these larvae is therefore much more important than recognition of the adults.

The first two species in the above list, *W. bancrofti* and *B, malayi*, with blood-inhabiting microfilariae, will be dealt with at some length. Then the remaining species will be dealt with relatively briefly, not because they are necessarily less important (indeed certain species like *Loa loa* and *Onchocerca volvulus* are of very great local importance), but because their life-cycles (so far as is known, and they are only partially known) and habits are similar in broad outline to those of *W. bancroft*, although the vectors are different. These remaining species may be divided into two groups: the first, in which the larvae, are blood-inhabiting, includes *Loa loa, Mansonella perstans* and *Mansonella ozzardi*; the second, in which the larvae do not normally occur in the blood but are found mainly in the lymph spaces in the skin, includes *Onchocerca volvulus* and *Mansonella streptocerca*.

Rarities like *Loa inquirenda* and *Dirofilaria magalhaesi* will not be dealt with because, like certain other filariae that have been recovered in man occasionally, they are probably normally parasitic in hosts other than man.

Wuchereria bancrofti

This helminth has a very wide distribution, mainly along the coastal belts of the tropics. It occurs in Africa, South America, China, Japan, Malaysia, Indonesia and the South Pacific. Its wide distribution, high infection rate and proved pathogenicity render it the most important of the filaria parasites of man.

The adult worms, both male and female, are found in tightly coiled masses in nodular dilatations of the lymphatic vessels and lymph glands, but wandering worms may occur in various other sites. The adult female measures about 8 cm in length and is threadlike, being only about 0.25 mm wide. The adult male measure about 3 cm. The posterior end is sharply coiled, and there are two unequal copulatory spicules.

The viviparous female in the lymphatic system discharges enormous numbers of larvae which find their way into the blood stream and appear in the peripheral circulation. They may be found in the blood at all hours of the day and night, but their numbers tend to increase from 9 p.m. onwards and to reach a maximum at about midnight; that is to say, the microfilariae of *W. bancrofti* exhibit nocturnal periodicity. In spite of much work, the phenomenon of periodicity has never been satisfactorily explained; but whatever the reason for the nocturnal increase, it is obviously well adapted to render night-biting insects the most suitable vectors for this parasite. In practice this is the case, and *W. bancrofti* is transmitted by species of mosquitoes that are mainly night-biting. In certain of the Pacific Islands east of longitude 180°E the fluctuation in numbers of microfilariae is relatively small, and here the vector is a day-biting mosquito, *Aedes variegatus*.

The microfilariae in the peripheral blood undergo no further development, and eventually perish, unless they are taken up by a suitable mosquito host. Complete development to the infective stage has been proved to take place in some 30-60 species of mosquitoes, and probably many more will allow this development. The important vectors vary in different parts of the world, and include species of *Culex, Aedes, Mansonia* and *Anopheles*.

Microfilariae that are taken up by a suitable mosquito develop in about 10 days to become infective larvae. There is no multiplication in the mosquito, one microfilaria giving rise to one infective larva, but the head of the infective mosquito may contain several larvae. When the mosquito again sucks blood from man, the infective larvae rupture through the proboscis, escape on to the skin and enter the tissues through a breach of the skin surface. The infective larvae are probably unable to penetrate unbroken skin.

Having penetrated the skin, the infective larvae migrate to the lymphatics and lymph glands, and in the course of 8–12 months become sexually mature adults. As the adult female lives in the lymphatics and not in the blood stream, the microfilariae, after birth, must reach the blood stream via the lymphatic ducts, thence to the venous system, and thence via the pulmonary capillaries to the peripheral circulation.

Brugia malayi

This parasite is very similar morphologically to *W. bancrofti*, and at one time was placed in the same genus. *Brugia* is found in many localities in India, South East Asia, Indonesia and the South Pacific, sometimes with *W. bancrofti* and sometimes alone. The adult male worm differs from *W. bancrofti* in that the posterior end of *B. malayi* is coiled on itself two to three times (once only in *W. bancrofti*), and that the spicules are slightly different. Both sexes are slightly smaller than those of *W. bancrofti*. The microfilariae also are smaller.

The development in the mosquito is similar to that of *W. bancrofti*. Microfilariae may appear in the blood of man as soon as 3 months after infection, as compared with 8–12 months for *W. bancrofti*. The lesions caused in man are similar to those caused by *W. bancrofti*, except that in *B. malayi* infections the elephantiasis nearly always involves the lower limbs and scrotal involvement does not occur.

Medical aspects of lymphatic filariasis

Pathogenesis

Pathological damage results from immune reactions of the host to adult and developing worms and their products within lymphatic tissues. Immune reactions are more likely to occur against damaged or dead worms than against healthy ones. Local trauma and chemotherapy may initiate immune processes by injuring worms. Immunoglobulin-E mast cell reactions, immune complex reactions and cell-mediated immunity reactions all take place.

In lymphatic tissue the results are recurrent acute inflammatory lymphadenitis and lymphangitis tending to recur at the same site for months or years. This is the inflammatory, early stage of filariasis. Sometimes abscess formation occurs. These painful attacks are difficult to differentiate from bacterial infections, but eosinophilia is often present.

In bancroftian filariasis the inguinal glands and lymphatics around the spermatic cord are often involved. Axillary, epitrochlear and retroperitoneal lymph glands may be inflamed; the latter condition is a diagnostic puzzle, mimicking pelvic sepsis. The acute inflammatory episodes usually last a few days and resolve spontaneously. There may be temporary lymphatic obstruction during these episodes, owing to endolymphangitis and causing distal pitting oedema of limbs or acute hydrocoele. *Brugia* infections are similar but rarely affect the genitalia. Many people infected with lymphatic filariasis are asymptomatic.

Late filariasis

In a minority (usually less than 5 per cent) of those infected, repeated attacks of lymphatic inflammation lead to fibrosis of lymphatics and permanent blockage with incompetent lymphatic valves below the block. Distal lymphoedema results, this becomes firm and non-pitting, and later there is hypertrophy of sub-cutaneous tissues with thickening, roughening and hyperkeratosis of the epithelium. This is 'elephantiasis'. Other sequelae of postinflammatory blockage include hydrocoele due to impaired lymphatic drainage from the tunica vaginalis, and lymph varices that are dilated, tortuous, thickened lymph vessels particularly found in the scrotum. Dilated lymph vessels in the scrotum may rupture externally, draining lymph from the scrotal skin so that the whole area is constantly damp and liable to bacterial infection. Rupture of dilated lymph vessels into the urinary system when there is a high abdominal lymphatic obstruction causes chyluria — the passage of milky chyle in the urine.

Elephantoid changes usually occur in the legs, but also appear in the scrotum and occasionally in arms and breasts. Elephantiasis is disabling, and affected tissues are very liable to recurrent bacterial infection, particularly with *Streptococcus pyogenes*.

Immunity

Adult worms succeed in avoiding immune destruction, although antibodies to adult worms are usually present in the serum. In cases with elephantiasis, micro-filariae are usually absent from the blood, and antibodies to the microfilariae are found in the blood. Some of those infected shows evidence of specific anti-filarial immune suppression by suppressor T-cells.

Clinical picture

Early inflammatory stages

Many of those infected are asymptomatic, as the severity of symptoms depends on the worm load and the host's immune responses. Symptoms usually appear 8–12 months after infection, but they can appear as early as 3 months. The initial symptom is usually the presence of a tender, hot swollen superficial lymph gland, often in the groin but sometimes in the axilla, the epitrochlear region or elsewhere. There is fever with systemic febrile symptoms — headache, joint and muscle pains. The patient is temporarily incapacitated until the painful episode ceases spontaneously after several days. Another common site of inflammation is the spermatic cord, causing funiculitis, and the testis, causing epididymo-orchitis often accompanied by a small acute hydrocoele. The spermatic cord is thickened, tender and sometimes irregularly beaded, particularly after recurrent attacks. Retroperitoneal lymphatic involvement causes acute abdominal pain and tenderness with fever. This may be confused with intra-abdominal sepsis, and indeed the condition may cause peritonitis. Abscess formation sometimes results from glandular inflammation.

Lymphadenitis may be associated with lymphangitis, appearing as a tender erythematous line or cord extending peripherally away from a lymph node, in contrast to lymphangitis resulting from skin sepsis which extends towards the draining node. Inflammatory synovitis of the knee joint is sometimes caused by *W. bancrofti*.

There may be a systemic febrile illness without localizing signs. This is probably due to involvement of a deep lymphatic gland, or an immune reaction to the moulting fluid of developing worms.

Recurrent inflammatory episodes, often in the same site, continue for months or years before ceasing. In a few of those infected, elephantiasis or other obstructive signs appear after 5–10 years. *Brugia* infections tend to advance to obstructive pathology more rapidly than do bancroftian infections, sometimes within 5 years.

Late obstructive lymphatic filariasis

Damage results from blockage of lymphatic fluid drainage. Hydrocoele is the commonest obstructive lesion in bancroftian filariasis, occurring to 10–20 per cent of those infected in some areas. Elephantiasis of the legs, often unilateral and confined to below the knee, occurs in up to 5 per cent of those infected. The surface of the limb is thickened and rough, with crevices between swollen areas. There may be warty excrescences on the feet. Elephantoid tissue is liable to recurrent attacks of bacterial infection, often due to haemolytic streptococci, and these infections cause further lymphatic damage. Scrotal elephantiasis is not uncommon, and may reach grotesque proportions with the mass of tissue weighing 20 kg or more. Fortunately the urethra is not obstructed. Elephantiasis of arms, breasts and vulva is less common. These masses of tissue are chronically disabling.

Dilated, tortuous lymph varices may be found in the scrotum and sub-cutaneously. Rupture of lymph vessels on to the skin causes maceration and bacterial infection. Chronic painless enlargement of lymph nodes, particularly in the groin, is another result of filariasis. Some patients have recurrent attacks of chyluria, passing milky urine. This may be preceded by back or abdominal pain and can be associated with haematuria. Usually chyluria is not serious; occasionally the loss of fat and protein in the urine is heavy and prolonged, leading to malnutrition.

Clinical diagnosis

The main problems in the inflammatory stages concern differentiation from bacterial infections. This can be difficult, and occasionally bacterial infections coexist with filarial ones. Eosinophilia and a history of recurrent episodes point to a filarial aetiology. Similar lymphatic obstructive lesions can be produced by other inflammatory and neoplastic lymphatic pathology. In Ethiopia, elephantiasis of the legs results from lymph node fibrosis caused by silicates,

Table 7.2 Differential diagnosis of lymphatic filariasis

Clinical presentation	Differential diagnosis	Diagnostic clues to filariasis
Painful lymphadenitis and lymphangitis; fever	Septic lesion of glands; lymphogranuloma venereum; plague	No primary skin lesion; centrifugal lymphatic spread; eosinophilia
Epididymo-orchitis; funiculitis	Gonococcal, bacterial and chlamydial epididymo-orchitis; torsion of testis	Absence of urethral discharge; presence of eosinophilia; microfilariae in acute hydrocoele fluid; thickened beaded spermatic cord; recurrent episodes
Chronic lymphadenopathy	Tuberculosis; reticulosis; onchocerciasis	History of inflammatory episodes; lymph node biopsy is avoided in filariasis — it increases obstruction
Elephantiasis	Lymphatic obstruction by TB; malignancy; silicates and chronic sepsis	History; positive serology for filariasis

presumably absorbed from the soles of the feet. Diagnostic problems are outlined in Table 7.2

Treatment of lymphatic filariasis

Specific
Diethylcarbamazine clears the circulation of microfilariae and has some action on adult worms; it is more effective in brugian than in bancroftian infections. There may be allergic reactions to dying worms during treatment, and lymph node abscesses occur, especially when treating *Brugia* infections. The usual dosage is 2 mg/kg 3 times a day for 3 weeks. Many advocate beginning with smaller doses, such as 1 mg/kg on day 1, 1 mg/kg 3 times on day 2, then 2 mg/kg 3 times a day for 19 days.

Levamisole and mebendazole have shown promise in treating *Brugia* infections.

Symptomatic and supportive
During acute inflammatory episodes the patient needs rest and analgesics such as paracetamol and aspirin. If the testis is involved, a scrotal supporting bandage is used. Specific chemotherapy is delayed until the acute episode has settled.

People who know they have a filarial infection fear elephantiasis — they should be reassured that this can be avoided by early treatment and is an unlikely outcome.

Late obstructive stage

Chemotherapy cannot reverse established elephantiasis, and management is often only palliative. Hydrocoele and elephantoid scrotum are treated surgically, but surgery for elephantoid limbs has not proved satisfactory. Supportive, firm bandaging of the leg before rising helps to control lymphoedema, and the technique of intermittent pneumatic compression is said to be of use. Because of the frequency of bacterial infection it is important to keep elephantoid tissue clean and dry. If there are recurrent haemolytic streptococcal infections, regular prophylactic penicillin is given as after rheumatic fever.

Medical aspects of tropical eosinophilia (occult filariasis)

Tropical eosinophilia is caused by a filarial infection with *W. bancrofti, B. malayi* or animal filarias in which there is an unusual immune response. The microfilariae are trapped in the tissues, surrounded by granulomas containing many eosinophils, and microfilariae are not found in the blood. Many of these granulomas are in the lungs, but they are also found in the liver and lymph glands. There is invariably a marked rise in eosinophils in the blood, to at least 3000, and sometimes as high as 50 000, per cubic millimetre.

Clinical features

The illness is found sporadically in endemic areas of filariasis, and appears most commonly in young Asian adults. There are usually respiratory symptoms, including cough, expectoration which is sometimes blood-stained, and dyspnoea with wheezing. Constitutional symptoms include low grade fever, lassitude and loss of weight. Crepitations and rhonchi may be heard on chest auscultation. Hepatomegaly, splenomegaly and a mild generalized lymphadenopathy may be found, sometimes without pulmonary symptoms. If untreated the disease continues for months, up to a year or more.

Changes in chest X-ray are seen in about 50 per cent of patients. These changes include miliary mottling and increased bronchial vascular markings. Spirometry often shows restrictive defects, and evidence of airways obstruction in some. Permanent pulmonary hypertension is a rare complication following treatment.

Diagnosis

Pulmonary tuberculosis, chronic bronchitis and asthma may all be confused with tropical eosinophilia. Larval pneumonitis due to ascariasis, hookworms and strongyloidiasis is much more transient. Pneumonitis due to toxocariasis may last some months.

Important points in the diagnosis of tropical eosinophilia are the invariably massive eosinophilia, strongly positive serological tests for filariasis without microfilariaemia, and prompt therapeutic response to diethylcarbamazine. Lung biopsy has been used in diagnosis, but it is rarely justifiable. A therapeutic trial of diethylcarbamazine is warranted in doubtful cases.

Treatment

The condition usually responds rapidly to diethylcarbamazine given in the doses recommended for bancroftian filariasis. Occasionally a second course of treatment is needed. Tetracycline can be used if diethylcarbamazine fails to cure.

Loa loa

This worm, because of its habit of making spasmodic appearances in the eye, was well known to early travellers in Africa at the beginning of the eighteenth century, and later in the century it was described by American workers who observed its presence in slaves imported to the New World. *Loa loa* has never become established outside Africa, where it is mainly confined to the tropical rain forest belt. It is particularly common in West Africa, but it also occurs in Central Africa and the Sudan.

The adults, male and female, are found in the mesentery, in the parietal peritoneum and under the skin. They are not uncommonly seen crossing the conjunctiva, and specimens from the living host are usually collected from this site, or from the abdomen during the course of surgical operations. The worms are long-lived and probably they can remain alive in the human host for as long as 15 years. Both males and females are thread-like, the males measuring about 3 cm and the females up to 7 cm.

The viviparous female during her wandering deposits the larvae in the tissue spaces, from where they reach the blood stream. The microfilariae exhibit a marked diurnal periodicity. The length of time for which the microfilariae can survive is not known, but they eventually perish unless taken up by the appropriate vector. The only known hosts that allow complete development of the larvae are flies of the genus *Chrysops*. The microfilariae taken up from the peripheral circulation develop in *Chrysops* in a very similar manner to the development of *W. bancrofti* in the mosquito. Development to the infective stage takes 10–14 days, at the end of which time the long filariform infective larvae accumulate in the head and proboscis of the fly; but unlike the infective forms of *W. bancrofti* they often migrate from the mouthparts to the abdomen, later returning to the head.

When an infective *Chrysops* again seeks a blood-meal, the larvae break out through the membrane at the base of the mouthparts and fall on the skin surface, often in very great numbers (as opposed to the few infective larvae of *W. bancrofti* from mosquitoes). The larvae probably require about a year to reach sexual maturity.

Medical aspects of loiasis

Pathogenesis and clinical manifestations

Some of those infected with *Loa loa* show no symptoms; many will have recurrent, transient subcutaneous swellings 10–20 cm in diameter lasting a few days and then resolving spontaneously. These swellings, known as 'Calabar swellings', are caused by allergic reactions to worm products released in the dermis. There may be mild general symptoms at the same time as the swellings. If near a joint such as the wrist, elbow or ankle there is joint pain with temporary swelling and loss of movement. Usually the lumps are mildly painful, somewhat itchy and slightly erythematous — pressure on a subcutaneous nerve produces more severe pain. Sometimes the worm crawls across the eye under the conjunctiva, where it is briefly visible. Ocular involvement does no permanent harm but it is painful, causes alarm in the patient, and produces local swelling which may close the eye for a day or two. The worms can live for 15 years, and these symptoms recur at irregular intervals (often of weeks or months) for many years. Although not usually causing serious harm, the lesions may be temporarily incapacitating. Sometimes worms can be seen under the skin without surrounding Calabar swellings.

Rarely, focal neurological syndromes occur as a result of ectopic worms in the brain. Acute encephalopathy with coma, and sometimes death, is a rare occurrence when heavily infected cases are treated with diethylcarbamazine. Presumably it is due to massive microfilarial destruction in the cerebral capillaries.

Treatment

Diethylcarbamazine is effective against adult worms, microfilariae and developing larvae. It is used in the doses recommended for treating bancroftian filariasis. Repeated courses may be needed. Heavily infected cases need careful supervision during treatment in case of development of encephalopathy, and such cases should start treatment with low doses of DEC as previously described, together with 1 mg/kg of prednisone daily for the first 7–10 days; exchange blood transfusion and plasmapheresis have also been advised, but these are usually impractical. Attempts to remove the worm surgically as it traverses the eye are unnecessary. Diethylcarbamazine acts on developing worms, and has shown activity as a prophylactic in dosage of 5 mg/kg on 3 consecutive days each month.

Mansonella perstans

This parasite is widely distributed in West, East and Central tropical Africa, and in the tropical regions of South America.

The adults are whitish; the female measures 7–8 cm in length and the male is about half this size. The tail in both sexes is distinctive, as it ends in two small triangular flaps. The male has two spicules, unequal in length.

The microfilariae of *M. perstans* are the smallest of the human microfilariae, and are easily recognized by this characteristics. They show no definite periodicity, but tend to be most numerous in the peripheral blood at night. The microfilariae are long-lived, and after experimental transfer to a host without adult worms they have remained alive for several years.

Development takes place in the midge *Culicoides*. The infective stage is reached after about 8 days' development in the midge.

M. perstans is generally recognized as non-pathogenic, but it is a common cause of symptomless eosinophilia.

Mansonella ozzardi

This species occurs only in the western hemisphere, in Central and South America and in the West Indies. The adult female measures 6–8 cm. Only one single incomplete male has been found in man, but specimens from monkeys are 2–3 cm long.

The microfilariae are almost as small as those of *M. perstans*. They show no periodicity. In experimental infections, the microfilariae will develop to the infective stage in particular species of *Culicoides* or of *Simulium*. Nothing is known of the time required for development in man from the infective stage to the adult.

M. ozzardi is generally considered to be non-pathogenic.

Mansonella streptocerca

This species is confined to West and Central Africa, and its range probably extends from Ghana to Zaire. It was for a long time known only by its micro-filariae, which resemble those of *M. perstans* but are longer and are found in the skin and not in the blood.

Only a few adults of *M. streptocerca* have been found, and the male has not been fully described. The adult female is about 27 mm long. The microfilariae appear in the skin, and they are unsheathed and non-periodic. The insect vector is *Culicoides grahamii*.

Infections are usually asymptomatic, but minor papular skin rashes may result. These are probably associated with cellular reactions to dead worms.

Onchocerca

The members of the genus *Onchocerca* are long, thread-like worms that live in the subcutaneous and connective tissues of their hosts, where many (but not all) of them are imprisoned in tough fibrous cysts or 'nodules'. The females are extremely long, and are usually so hopelessly entangled in the nodular tissue that it is very difficult to obtain entire specimens. In man, the females often reach a length of over 50 cm; in cattle they reach twice this length or even more. The males are comparatively small, about 2–5 cm long and 200 μm thick. The microfilariae are pointed-tailed and unsheathed, and do not normally enter the blood stream but stay in the skin and eye tissues.

A number of species have been described from horses, cattle, antelopes and man, but they are very difficult to distinguish — in some cases they have been distinguished mainly on the basis of the usual location of the nodules on the host's body. All species have thickened ridge-like rings on the cuticle, much more conspicuous in the females than in the males. The male has a coiled tail, bluntly rounded at the tip, and two unequal spicules. The females have a bluntly rounded tail.

Some species, especially *O. gibsoni*, injure the hides and carcasses of cattle by the hard nodules that form. Others, such as *O. reticulata*, cause papular, itching sores in horses. The intermediate hosts of the species of *Onchocerca* found in cattle and horses are species of *Culicoides* and *Simulium*.

Human onchocerciasis is caused by *O. volvulus*, which is widespread in

Equatorial Africa and Central and South America; there is also a small focus in Yemen and Saudi Arabia. *O. volvulus* was probably originally an African infection, and has been introduced rather recently into Central America, where it was not discovered until 1915. In some localities over 80 per cent of people harbour this worm, and 5 per cent of them lose their sight.

The developing worms creep about in the subcutaneous tissue, but when they finally pair and come to rest there is an inflammatory reaction that results in the formation of the characteristic fibrous cyst. A nodule has been found in a child two months old, but usually a much longer time is taken for them to appear. Nodules may grow to a diameter of 1 cm in a year, but usually the rate of growth is slower. In America there seem usually to be a few (3 or 4) worms in a cyst, but in Africa composite nodules have been found containing over 100 worms.

The worms lie in tangles in the cyst, which vary from the size of a pea or even smaller to that of a pigeon's egg. Usually there is also a swarm of microfilariae in the cyst. In most localities infected people have only a few nodules, but in some places in Africa 25–100 nodules are commonly seen, most of them only a few millimetres in diameter. There is ample evidence, however, that not all the adult worms become encapsulated.

The intermediate host is *Simulium*. The microfilariae in the skin are taken up by the biting fly, and development takes place mainly in the thoracic muscles, as with the other filariae. Infective larvae are produced within about 7 days of the fly's feeding.

Medical aspects of onchocerciasis

Pathogenesis

Pathological damage in onchocerciasis results from immune reactions to dead or damaged microfilariae. In the skin the microfilariae are usually situated just under the epithelium; if they are alive there is often no clear reaction to them, but if they are damaged there is local cellular infiltration, oedema and pigmentary changes. This inflammatory process is exaggerated when microfilaricidal drugs such as diethylcarbamazine are given — microfilariae migrate into the epithelium, and epithelial microabscesses are formed and give rise to itchy papules. Subacute inflammatory changes gradually give way to dermal fibrosis and atrophy. Skin damage is increased by scratching, which causes lichenification and secondary bacterial infection. Some of the adult worms are surrounded by fibrous capsules and lie in subcutaneous nodules. In Africa these nodules are often found over bony prominences on the leg, such as trochanters and epicondyles of the knees and around the iliac crests, on the sides of the chest wall and scapular regions. Although unsightly and uncomfortable to lie on, these nodules cause no serious damage. In America the nodules are often found on the head.

Groups of lymphatic glands are often enlarged owing to local cell-mediated immunity, with immune complex Arthus-type reactions around dead microfilariae. Nodes in the inguinal-femoral region are commonly enlarged; rarely lymphatic obstruction may result, causing scrotal or leg elephantiasis.

In heavy infections all parts of the eye may be invaded by microfilariae, which on dying produce inflammatory reactions. The extent of ocular damage depends on the number of microfilariae present, the duration of infection, whether the infection is in forest or savannah, and reactions to chemotherapy. Early infections cause superficial inflammation to the cornea (superficial keratitis). In heavy infections sclerosing keratitis with eventual pupillary opacification, iritis and glaucoma leads to blindness. Retinal lesions also occur, causing choroidoretinitis and optic atrophy.

Heavy onchocercal infections are associated with a lower than average height/weight ratio, diminished life expectancy and some degree of immunosuppression which renders subjects more likely to lepromatous leprosy. Damaging immune reactions occur in eye and skin in response to rapid massive microfilarial destruction by diethylcarbamazine (the 'Mazzotti reaction').

A general picture emerges of a gradual build-up of parasite load over many years, with slowly progressive skin and eye damage — inflammation, fibrosis and atrophy.

Skin changes

Some of those infected show no symptoms even though skin snips show large numbers of microfilariae. The commonest symptom is itching, even before cutaneous lesions appear. The earliest skin changes in dark skins are areas of hyperpigmentation, often over the femoral trochanters. Later there may be papular rashes, excoriations, and sometimes quite acute oedema of skin. Partly as a response to scratching, parts of the skin become roughened and thickened (lichenification). Eventually, after years, the skin becomes thin, atrophic, wrinkled and prematurely aged, particularly in the lower parts of the body. There is also patchy depigmentation over the shins, known as 'leopard skin' because of its spotted appearance. Nodules are smooth, round, non-tender, usually mobile subcutaneous lumps 0.5–5 cm or more in diameter. They tend to occur in small groups over bony prominences, such as the femoral trochanters, iliac crests, epicondyles of the knees and sacrum in Africans, and on the head in American onchocerciasis.

A moderate generalized lymphadenopathy, most obvious in the inguino-femoral region, is common. Marked inguinal lymphadenopathy covered by atrophic baggy skin in the groins may hang down in the inguinal region, when the condition is known as 'hanging groin'. It predisposes to hernia formation.

In the Yemen there is an unusual variety of onchocerciasis known as Sowda (Arabic = black). Usually one leg is involved, the skin is very dark and thickened, and the inguinal glands are large and fleshy (histologically a humoral immune type of response).

Elephantiasis of leg or scrotum is an unusual manifestation of onchocerciasis.

Expatriates often respond vigorously to light infections, with severe itching and erythematous papules sometimes confined to one or both buttocks and thighs.

Eye changes

Early symptoms of eye damage include itching and irritation of the eyes. Later there may be watering of the eyes, photophobia, poor nocturnal vision and then deteriorating vision.

The cornea shows small white areas (snowflake opacities) of inflammation around dead microfilariae. Later, scarring keratitis encroaches on the lateral and inferior margins of the cornea, eventually causing scarring and opacification.

On examination with a slit lamp, living active coiled microfilariae may be seen in the anterior chamber of the eye. Iritis with pigmentary changes, posterior synechiae and pupil irregularity also occur, and may lead to glaucoma and blindness. Retinal changes include choroidoretinitis with pigmentation, retinal atrophy and optic atrophy.

Clinical diagnosis

Onchocerciasis needs consideration in pruritus, skin rashes, subcutaneous nodules and eye problems in endemic areas. Scabies is a common cause of pruritus and papular rashes in the tropics, and typical burrows should be sought on wrists and finger webs.

Treatment

Treatment of onchocerciasis has proved difficult because diethylcarbamazine destroys microfilaria but not adult worms, and it provokes intense inflammatory activity in relation to the massive destruction of microfilariae. This reaction to diethylcarbamazine is known as the Mazzotti reaction, and is manifested by the onset of severe itching, often with papular rashes, swelling and pain in enlarged inguinal lymph nodes, fever and hypotension. The Mazzotti reaction usually starts within an hour or two of drug administration, and may last for several days. In a few heavily infected feeble patients it has caused death. There may be painful, sterile effusions into joints a week or so later, suggestive of immune complex reactions. Attempts to diminish Mazzotti reactions with antihistamines and serotonin antagonists have not been successful. Steroids diminish some aspects of the Mazzotti reaction but lessen the microfilaricidal action. In the heavily infected eye Mazzotti reactions can cause severe inflammation with permanent damage and visual loss; local corticosteroid drugs diminish inflammatory changes in the eyes.

Diethylcarbamazine should be used with caution in onchocerciasis, beginning with a schedule such as: day 1, 25 mg twice daily; day 2, 50 mg twice daily; day 3, 100 mg twice daily; day 4–21, 200 mg 3 times a day. Awadzi in Ghana has achieved over 90 per cent microfilariae destruction with a schedule of 50 mg daily for 2 days, followed by 100 mg twice daily for 14 days.

Aspirin or paracetamol is used as symptomatic treatment for the Mazzotti reaction. Diethylcarbamazine is temporarily stopped and restarted gradually if the reaction is severe. It is probably wisest not to use diethylcarbamazine in people with anything but very early eye involvement.

Suramin
This is a complex organic substance, a derivative of the trypan dyes, which is administered intravenously, binds strongly to plasma proteins, and has a very long half-life in the body. It has a macrofilaricidal action and a slow microfilaricidal action. The usual recommended dose is a test dose of 200 mg by slow intra-

venous injection to detect the occasional hypersensitivity reaction, followed by 1 g at weekly intervals for 5 weeks. Recently it has been suggested that lower dosages totalling 4.2 g (0.4, 0.4, 0.6, 0.8, 1.0, 1.0 g weekly) are effective and safer. Unfortunately suramin may cause serious toxic reactions. An immediate hypersensitivity reaction with nausea, vomiting and shock occurs rarely, in about 1 in 500 patients. Abdominal pain and urticaria sometimes follow injection. Papular eruptions and hyperaesthesia of hands and soles of the feet may occur and presage peripheral neuritis. More seriously renal damage is sometimes found; traces of albuminuria are common but heavier albuminuria should lead to cessation of treatment. The urine must be tested for albumin before each injection. Delayed but prolonged Mazzotti reactions are sometimes seen after suramin treatment. Rarely a serious, sometimes fatal, wasting illness with oral ulceration and diarrhoea occurs; exfoliative dermatitis can cause serious illness. Suramin is safer to use than diethylcarbamazine if the eyes are involved to any extent.

The effect of diethylcarbamazine alone in onchocerciasis is temporary, as the adult worms are not affected and continue to produce larvae. Diethylcarbamazine treatment should therefore be followed by a course of suramin.

Recently ivermectin in one single oral dose of 100–200 μg/kg has shown considerable promise as a microfilaricide, destroying microfilariae without causing severe Mazzotti reactions or eye problems. Metrifonate and mebendazole combined with levamisole have microfilaricidal action, but they do cause Mazzotti reactions (though often less severe than those caused by diethylcarbamazine) and have no real advantage.

Nodulectomy
Removal of nodules does eliminate some of the adult worms, but many worms exist outside nodules, and some nodules are clinically undetectable. Nodulectomy has been used with some success in South America, when nodules have been removed from the head, and it may have helped to prevent blindness in these cases. It is not considered to be a very efficient or cost-effective therapeutic procedure.

Superfamily Dracunculoidea

These worms were once included with the filarias, but members of the Dracunculoidea are peculiar in the relatively enormous size of the female, as compared with the midget male, and in the fact that during the course of their development the alimentary canal and the vulva atrophy, leaving the body of the female almost entirely occupied by the embryo-filled uterus. The embryos are liberated by the bursting of a loop of the uterus prolapsed through the mouth or through a rupture of the anterior end of the body. The worms in this group are all parasites living in the tissues of vertebrates. Only one species, *Dracunculus medinensis*, is known to parasitize man.

Dracunculus medinensis

The cause of the disease dracunculiasis or dracontiasis is often called the dragon worm or the serpent worm, but its most common name is the guinea worm.

Written descriptions of this parasite are among the earliest known. At one time *D. medinensis* was confined to the Old World, but it has now spread to the New World, almost certainly as a result of the slave trade. At present it is mainly a parasite of Africa and India.

D. medinensis is usually considered only to infect man, but other (and similar) species have been recorded from various domestic animals (dogs in particular) and from the raccoon and mink. Whether the species found in these animals are transmissible to man is not known, but in any case there does not seem to be a normal animal reservoir for the human infection.

The adult female worms are found in the subcutaneous tissues of man. On average they measure about 80 cm in length and are thread-like, being only about 2 mm in diameter. The tail is curved to form a hook, similar to that often seen in male nematodes, and probably the female is anchored in the host tissue by the hooked tail. In the gravid female the gut is atrophied and the body cavity is almost completely filled by the coiled uterus packed with larvae. The male is about 4 cm long, and has a spirally coiled tail. It is rarely seen, and only a few specimens have been recovered from man.

The life-cycle of the guinea worm is unlike that of any other helminth that parasitizes man. Fertilization of the female probably takes place in the deep connective tissues of the host, and afterwards the female migrates to the subcutaneous tissues in almost any part of the body — although 90 per cent of the worms are found in the lower limbs, generally below knee level.

Having reached the final site, where its outline can sometimes be seen (or, more often, felt), the worm stimulates the formation of a blister in the overlying skin. Sooner or later this blister bursts, exposing a shallow ulcer with the head of the worm in the centre. If this ulcer comes into contact with water at a temperature lower than the skin, the worm responds to the stimulus by protruding a coil of uterus which ruptures and discharges a puff of milky fluid, clearly visible to the naked eye, into the surrounding water. This fluid contains large numbers of coiled larvae about 600 μm long (Fig. 7.2). After an hour or so the worm is ready to discharge another brood of larvae, and this process continues throughout the worm's remaining life. Usually the worm lives 2–3 weeks, but it may live considerably longer. Finally the female worm dies and is absorbed into the host tissue, but occasionally it emerges spontaneously.

In suitably muddy water the larvae may remain alive for some weeks, but if by the end of this time they have not gained access to a suitable intermediate host they die. The larvae develop further if they are ingested by a suitable crustacean, such as *Cyclops*. The ingested larvae grow in the body cavity of the crustacean, and after about 2 weeks become infective third-stage larvae. The developing larvae, although they do not kill the crustacean, render it less active, so that in still water such as in wells the infected crustaceans tend to accumulate at the bottom while the uninfected and more active ones inhabit the upper zones.

If the infected crustaceans are ingested by man they are at once destroyed in the stomach, but the released infective larvae bore into the host tissues. Their subsequent development to the adult stage probably requires about 6 months, but the gravid females seldom appear in their final subcutaneous site until about 12 months after the ingestion of the infective larvae.

Medical aspects of dracunculiasis

Pathogenesis

Guinea worms cause no symptoms until a few days before emergence through the skin. Then there may be symptoms suggestive of a systemic hypersensitivity illness with urticaria, periorbital oedema, wheezing, hypotension and vomiting. These symptoms are due to allergic host reactions to liberation of worm secretions into the tissues. Substances secreted at the site of emergence cause subcutaneous inflammation and local blister formation. This itchy painful blister ruptures or is scratched open and an ulcer results. The worm's uterus penetrates the body of the worm and prolapses into the ulcer, discharging its larvae. The ulcer is liable to secondary infection, causing spreading cellulitis, septic arthritis of nearby joints, especially the ankle, and tetanus. Local and general allergic symptoms arise if the worm is ruptured during attempted extraction. Usually all the embryos are discharged in 3–4 weeks; then the worm dies and is reabsorbed, extruded or calcified. Following death of the worm, the ulcer will heal if secondary sepsis is dealt with.

Immunity to reinfection is poor; some people have recurrent infections for many years.

Clinical manifestations

The incubation period is about a year. The worm is sometimes visible under the skin but causes no symptoms until a few days before emergence, when the general allergic symptoms described above may appear. Local pain and irritation precede the appearance and rupture of the blister, which is usually on the lower leg but can be on other parts of the body. The resultant ulcer usually becomes infected with bacteria, causing local pain, cellulitis, joint involvement and sometimes tetanus. Septic arthritis and ankylosis of the ankle may follow. Local swelling and pain as well as general allergic symptoms occur if the worm is ruptured during attempts at extraction. Rarely the female worm lodges in the spinal canal, compresses the spinal cord, and causes paraplegia.

Guinea worm infection is very prevalent in some village communities. It is temporarily disabling and sometimes causes serious or fatal illness, and it is a serious public health problem in some areas.

Diagnosis

There is usually little doubt about the diagnosis if the head of the worm is seen in the ulcer. Application of cold water results in a milky discharge of myriads of larvae which can be identified under a microscope. Other common causes of ulcers in the tropics are listed on p. 73.

Management

It is important to keep the ulcer clean and covered. Moist dressings may accelerate larval discharge and shorten the illness. Secondary infections must be treated with antibiotics, and appropriate tetanus prophylaxis administered.

The traditional treatment is gradual, gentle extraction by winding the worm onto a small stick. A few centimetres only are extracted daily, and impatience leads to rupture of the worm with serious local and general symptoms. Metronidazole 200 mg 3 times a day for 7 days, or niridazole 25 mg/kg daily in 3 divided doses for 7 days, facilitates worm removal. The drugs probably act by reducing local inflammation rather than by killing the worm.

Laboratory identification of nematodes

Adult or larval nematodes may be found in the faeces, particularly after purges, or in the subcutaneous tissues of man. Usually, however, infections with nematode parasites of the alimentary canal are identified by finding characteristic eggs in the faeces, and infections with nematode parasites of the lymphatic system and connective tissue (the filarias) are identified by finding the characteristic larvae in the blood or skin.

Identification of eggs

The eggs of nematode parasites of the alimentary canal of man are on the whole readily identifiable, although the eggs of the two species of hookworms are practically indistinguishable.

Ascaris lumbricoides eggs

The fertile eggs are spherical or ovoid in shape, and about 60 μm long and 45 μm wide. The very thick clear egg shell is covered by an irregular albuminous coat, which is usually a golden-brown colour. The egg contains a very conspicuous unsegmented fertilized ovum which is contracted away from the poles (Fig. 9.2).

Unfertilized eggs are frequently seen in faeces. They are sometimes passed because the host harbours only female worms, but are more often passed by fertilized females in the early stages of oviposition. These eggs are more elongated than fertile eggs (sometimes as long as 90 μm), have a thinner shell, and frequently a thinner albuminous coating. The colour is similar to that of the fertile eggs, but the ovum is unorganized and appears as a mass of refractile granules (Fig. 9.2).

Occasionally the albuminous coating of *Ascaris* eggs is lost, altering the characteristic appearance and making the eggs difficult to recognize. Decorticated eggs can be identified by the thick shell and the large unsegmented ovum (Fig. 9.2). Decorticated infertile eggs are irregular in shape and have a thinner shell, and may be confused with certain other nematode eggs or with plant cells. However, decorticated eggs do not occur in faeces without normal corticated eggs being present.

Enterobius vermicularis eggs

The eggs are colourless, basically an elongate ovoid but flattened on one side, with a fairly thick shell, and about 55 μm long and 25 μm wide (Fig. 9.2). When passed they contain a tadpole-shaped larva. *Enterobius* does not usually lay eggs in the intestine. The gravid female worm migrates to the rectum, and during the night passes through the anus and deposits eggs on the perianal skin. Eggs are therefore only occasionally found in the faeces, and are usually collected by applying sticky transparent tape to the perianal skin.

Trichuris trichiura eggs

The eggs are brown, barrel-shaped, with a conspicuous colourless polar plug protruding from each end, and about 50 μm long and 25 μm wide (Fig. 9.2). When passed in faeces the egg contains a large unsegmented ovum.

Capillaria philippensis eggs

The eggs are rather like *Trichuris* eggs, but they have a pitted shell, they are parallel-sided rather than barrel-shaped, and the polar plugs do not protrude. They are about 45 μm long and 20 μm wide (Fig. 7.2).

Ancylostoma duodenale and *Necator americanus*

The eggs of the two species of hookworm infecting man are practically indistinguishable. They are oval and colourless, with bluntly rounded ends and a very thin egg shell, and about 60 μm long and 40 μm wide (Fig. 9.2). The egg of *Necator* has been described as being longer (about 70 μm) and very slightly narrower, but the differences between the two species are too small to be used for diagnostic purposes. When passed in the faeces the egg usually contains an ovum that has divided into two, four or eight cells. There is an obvious clear space between the egg shell and the segmented ovum.

Identification of microfilariae

The adults of the seven species of filarial worm that commonly infect man can be distinguished morphologically, but as these adults are obtained only during post-mortem examinations or surgical operations, diagnosis is usually based on an examination of microfilariae found in the blood or skin. The following are the characters most frequently used for establishing the identity of the different species of microfilariae.

Habitat

Most species of microfilariae appear in the peripheral blood, but some are found only in the skin or in the subcutaneous tissue. The habitat of the larvae is associated with the biting habits of the vector. Where the microfilariae occur in the blood they are transmitted by files which tap the capillaries without obvious laceration of the cuticle, but where the microfilariae are absent from the blood and appear only in the skin they are transmitted by flies which have mouthparts adapted to rasping the skin before reaching the capillaries.

Periodicity

Certain species of blood-inhabiting microfilariae appear in the peripheral circulation in greatest numbers during the day (diurnal periodicity), others in greatest numbers at night (nocturnal periodicity), and others show no such variation in numbers and are said to exhibit no periodicity, or to be aperiodic. In some strains of *W. bancrofti* and *B. malayi* the peak in intensity of microfilariae is not very marked, and these strains are sometimes referred to as being subperiodic. The periodicity is related to the habits of the insect vector. Usually microfilariae with diurnal periodicity are transmitted by day-biting flies, while those with nocturnal periodicity are transmitted by night-biting flies.

Presence or absence of a sheath

Certain species of microfilariae possess an outer covering or 'sheath' which they normally retain until after ingestion by the insect vector. The sheath fits the larva very closely in its lateral aspect, but it is considerably longer than the body and in fresh preparations can sometimes be seen projecting at one end or both ends. The sheath can be seen in preparations stained with haemalum, and may be seen in preparations stained with Giemsa's stain. The origin of the sheath is not known, but it seems probable that when the larva hatches from the egg it fails to rupture the fine (but very strong) vitelline membrane, and carries this membrane with it.

Arrangement of the column of nuclei

The microfilariae seen in the vertebrate host are without a gut, but the future position of the gut is marked by a column of cells that stand out prominently in suitably stained preparations. This column of cells shows certain breaks or gaps, but has a uniform pattern within the different species. For identification of the microfilariae found in man, however, it is necessary only to examine the nuclei at the tail end and to note their relative size and shape, whether they are single or double, and how close they extend to the tip of the tail. Other points of morphology of importance are the length of the microfilariae, the regularity or otherwise of the body curves in a stained blood film, and the shape and curvature of the tail.

The microfilariae found in man can be identified by the following characteristics.

Wuchereria bancrofti

The microfilariae are blood-inhabiting. They may be found in the blood at any time of the day or night, but their numbers tend to increase from 21.00 hours onwards and to reach a maximum about midnight; that is to say, the microfilariae exhibit nocturnal periodicity. (Certain strains found in the Pacific Islands are diurnally sub-periodic.) The microfilariae are about 250–300 μm long and are actively motile, so that their presence in the blood can be easily recognized with a low-power microscope. The microfilariae are sheathed. The sheath shows clearly when stained with haemalum, but does not normally show in blood films stained with Giemsa's stain. In dried blood films the microfilariae usually lie in smooth graceful curves. The nuclei do not extend to the tip of the tail (Fig. 7.3).

Sheathed, in blood

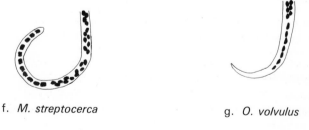

a. *W. bancrofti*   b. *B. malayi*   c. *L. loa*

Unsheathed, in blood

d. *M. ozzardi*   e. *M. perstans*

Unsheathed, in skin

f. *M. streptocerca*   g. *O. volvulus*

Fig. 7.3 Arrangement of nuclei in tails of microfilariae. *Sheathed, in blood*: a. *W. bancrofti*; b. *B. malayi*; c. *L. loa*.
Unsheathed, in blood: d. *M. ozzardi*; e. *M. perstans*.
Unsheathed, in skin: f. *M. streptocerca*; g. *O. volvulus*.

Brugia malayi

The microfilariae are blood-inhabiting, and show a nocturnal periodicity. (Some strains found in parts of Malaysia, Borneo, Thailand and the Philippines are sub-periodic.) The microfilariae are slightly smaller than those of *W. bancrofti*, being up to 230 μm long and are sheathed. The sheath stains with haemalum, and stains pink with Giemsa's stain. In dried blood films the microfilariae do not lie in smooth curves, but show secondary kinks. The tip of the tail of the microfilaria has two small distinct nuclei in a clear space in a terminal thread (Fig. 7.3).

Loa loa

The microfilariae are blood-inhabiting, and show a diurnal periodicity. They are sheathed, and about 250–300 μm long. The sheath stains clearly with haemalum, but does not stain with Giemsa's stain. (When stained with Giemsa's stain, however, the genital cells of the microfilariae stain a deep pink.) In dried blood films the microfilariae usually have a twisted appearance, and the tail is often doubled back along the body. The column of nuclei extends to the tip of the tail (Fig. 7.3).

Mansonella perstans

The microfilariae are blood-inhabiting and aperiodic. They are unsheathed, and about 100 μm long. In dried blood films they frequently lie in a coil. The double column of nuclei extends to the tip of the tail (Fig. 7.3).

Mansonella ozzardi

The microfilariae are blood-inhabiting and aperiodic. They are unsheathed and about 200 μm long. The column of nuclei does not extend to the tip of the tail (Fig. 7.3).

Mansonella streptocerca

The microfilariae are skin-inhabiting, aperiodic and unsheathed. They are about 150–200 μm long, and the single column of nuclei extends to the tip of the tail. In dried films the tail of the microfilariae if frequently crooked (Fig. 7.3).

Onchocerca volvulus

The microfilariae are skin-inhabiting, aperiodic and unsheathed. They are about 250–300 μm long, and the single column of nuclei does not extend to the tip of the tail (Fig. 7.3).

Identification of other stages

Certain of the nematode parasites of man cannot be identified by the finding of eggs or microfilariae, and identification of these parasites requires the recognition of other stages in the life-cycle.

Trichinella spiralis

Laboratory diagnosis of trichinosis depends on the finding of encysted larvae in muscle tissue obtained by biopsy. The muscle may be artificially digested to release the larvae, or simply crushed between two glass plates and examined microscopically for encysted larvae. The cysts are lemon-shaped, about 500 μm long and 200 μm wide, and each may contain several larvae (Fig. 7.2).

Strongyloides stercoralis

The eggs of *Strongyloides* usually hatch in the intestine immediately they are laid, so that only larvae appear in the faeces. The larvae are about 250 μm long when they hatch, but may be as long as 400 μm when they appear in the faeces (Fig. 7.2). These larvae are similar to hookworm larvae, but can be distinguished because they are present in freshly passed faeces, and because the length of the buccal cavity is about one-third the width of the head (in hookworm larvae it is about equal to the width of the head).

Dracunculus medinensis

Diagnosis is usually by finding the adult worm in an ulcer at the skin surface on medical examination. If a drop of water is left on the ulcer for a few minutes and then transferred to a microscope slide, the characteristic larvae will usually be seen. The larvae are about 500–700 μm long, with a rounded anterior and a long, tapering, sharply pointed tail occupying about one-third of the total length of the larvae (Fig. 7.2). Unlike the microfilariae, the larvae of *Dracunculus* have a clearly defined oesophagus and gut. In water they swim by alternately coiling and uncoiling.

Visceral larva migrans

The diagnosis of visceral larva migrans must be based on clinical symptoms (which are not specific) combined with the presence of eosinophilia with no other signs of parasitic infection, or on serological tests, which are not highly specific.

Cutaneous larva migrans

Diagnosis depends on observing the characteristic shape of the sinuous larvae moving in the subcutaneous tissues.

The principles of control of soil-transmitted nematodes

The importance of a general improvement in hygienic and socio-economic conditions is the same as for the control of intestinal protozoa (see end of Chapter 1). Health education concerning the mode of spread and the prevention of these diseases, and the provision and use of suitable latrines, are of fundamental importance.

Ascaris and *Trichuris* infections

These infections are spread by the faeco-oral route, usually by ingestion of infective eggs on vegetables or fruits that grow on or near the ground. These should not be eaten raw but should be peeled or cooked as appropriate. Human faeces which are used as manure are a source of infection. Storage or composting of faeces for 8 weeks is usually sufficient to ensure that most contained helminth eggs are non-infective.

Children may be infected by putting soil-contaminated fingers or other objects in their mouths. It is difficult to prevent this, but efforts must be made to stop their indiscriminate defaecation outside. Mass treatment of *Ascaris* infections has been successful in some areas; it needs to be repeated until the transmission rate is low enough to prevent widespread infection. Initially treatment may need to be repeated two or three times a year. If transmission is seasonal, treatment schedules should begin a month before the expected onset of transmission and continue until 2 months after its end. Levamisole in a single dose of 4 mg/kg is a suitable drug to use.

Hookworm and *Strongyloides* infections

Infection is by larvae penetrating the skin, so proper disposal of faeces is essential for control. Pit or borehole latrines are needed. Burying faeces with a trowel has been suggested for farmers defaecating in the fields, but such burying may not be deep enough as hookworm larvae are said to be capable of climbing 90 cm upwards through the soil. Theoretically the wearing of shoes should diminish infection, but this precaution has never proved very successful in practice.

Mass treatment campaigns, which often need repetition, have had some success when combined with the provision of latrines. Reduction of the worm loads will lower the incidence of disease due to hookworms even though the parasite is not eliminated.

Toxocariasis

Prevention of this infection depends on repeated deworming of dogs and puppies. It is impossible to control the fouling of public places by dogs. Some would advocate that young children should not have contact with puppies.

Control of lymphatic filariasis

Control of lymphatic filariasis has largely depended on mass treatment and vector control. Elimination of the parasites from a human population has proved very difficult, but marked reduction of the worm loads has achieved considerable lessening of the incidence of inflammatory and obstructive disease. Diethylcarbamazine is the only suitable drug for mass treatment — and it is often used at a dosage of 6 mg/kg in one dose monthly for 12 months. There may be marked allergic reactions in some patients, showing as fever, body pains and lymphadenitis. These reactions are more severe in *B. malayi* infections than in *W. bancrofti* infections.

Control of the vectors of filariasis is often difficult. Where anopheline mosquitoes are the principal vectors, as in parts of East Africa, antimalarial spraying considerably reduces transmission of filariasis. In contrast *Culex quinquefasciatus*, an important vector of filariasis in urban areas in Asia, breeds abundantly in many peridomestic sites and is resistant to many insecticides. Its control has proved very difficult, and filariasis has increased in many urban areas. *Aedes* control, by the use of spraying techniques and controlling breeding sites, has been rather more successful. Control of *Mansonoides* mosquitoes in rural areas of South East Asia has also been difficult, and in addition there are problems caused by the existence of an animal reservoir in monkeys and other wild animals. This has made the control of subperiodic *B. malayi* filariasis very difficult.

Mass treatment campaigns have proved more successful than vector control, but all control methods should be used in combination. Screening of houses against mosquitoes and the use of bed nets have parts to play in control programmes.

Control of onchocerciasis

Vector control is the main measure used to control onchocerciasis. This control has depended on dosing the riverine breeding sites of *Simulium* with insecticides. In the Volta basin in West Africa the WHO has begun a control operation on a huge scale using the organo-phosphate Temephos (Abate) sprayed from helicopters. This has freed large areas from *S. damnosum* and stopped transmission of onchocerciasis in these areas; but there are now reports of resistance to Temephos, and of reinvasion of treated areas by *Simulium* flies travelling long distances of up to 300 km. Because of the long life of *O. volvulus*, it is planned to continue control operations for twenty years. The vector of O. volvulus in Kenya, *S. neavei*, was successfully dealt with by the application of DDT to the rivers where *S. neavei* bred.

There is at the moment no suitable drug for the mass treatment of onchocerciasis, but the potentialities of ivermectin are promising. Nodulectomy has had some effect in preventing blindness in South America, but it is not an efficient general control measure.

Further reading

Banwell JG, Shad GA. Hookworm. *Clin Gastroenterol* 1978; **7**: 129–56.
Buck AA. (ed). **1974** *Onchocerciasis: Symptomatology, Pathology and Diagnosis.* Geneva, World Health Organization 1974.
Denham DA, McGreevy PB. 1977 Brugian filariasis: epidemiological and experimental studies. *Adv in Parasitol* 1977; **15**: 243–309.
Filho EC. Strongyloidiasis. *Clin in Gastroenterol* 1978; **7**: 179–200.
Miller TA. Hookworm infection in man. *Adv Parasitol* 1979; **17**: 315–84.
Most H. Trichinosis — preventable yet still with us. *New Engl J Med* 1978; **298**: 1178–80.
Muller R. Guinea worm disease: epidemiology, control and treatment. *Bull World Health Organization* 1979; **57**: 683–689.
Pawlowski ZS. Ascariasis. *Clin Gastroenterol* 1978; **7**: 157–78.
Sasa M. Human filariasis. University Park Press, Baltimore. 1976.

Watten RH, Beckner WH, Cross JH, Gunning J-J, Jaramillo J. Clinical studies of capillariasis phillippinensis. *Trans Roy Soc Tropical Med* Hyg 1972; **66**: 828–34.

Wolfe MS. *Oxyuris, trichostrongylus* and *trichuris*. *Clin Gastroenterol* 1978; **7**: 201–217.

W.H.O. Intestinal, Protozoan and Helminthic Infections. Geneva: WHO Technical Report Series 666, 1981.

W.H.O. *Epidemiology of onchocerciasis*. Geneva: WHO Technical Report Series 597, 1976.

Part III

Laboratory diagnostic techniques

Very few of the parasitic diseases of man can be diagnosed on clinical grounds without the aid of information from laboratory investigations. While it is true that an indication — possibly a very good indication — of the cause of the disease may be obtained from clinical examination coupled with the geographical and medical history of the patient, the clinical signs of parasitic disease are rarely specific. A practitioner who has some knowledge of parasitological techniques may, however, be able to make a diagnosis on definite parasitic findings, or alternatively satisfy himself that the disease is not of parasitic origin. In either of these cases treatment can be given confidently, whereas it can only be given with uncertainty when the real cause of the condition is not known.

Even when technical assistance is available, knowledge of the relevant diagnostic methods enables the practitioner to check and confirm the laboratory findings if he wishes to do so. More importantly, the practitioner who has learned the necessary techniques can make the required preparations and examine them for parasites in emergencies when assistance may not be available; and treatment may then be commenced earlier than might otherwise have been possible.

The presence in man of most of the parasites described in this book can be recognized by the microscopical examination of smears of faeces or films of blood (or occasionally of other body fluids). The techniques for making smears of films can be learned relatively easily but good preparations are extremely important. Once the smears or films are made, they can be examined by basically simple techniques that require only common laboratory equipment, a few simple stains and reagents, and a microscope. These techniques, which are described in the following chapters, should be adequate for diagnosing most parasitic infections. However, for some infections it may be necessary to employ more elaborate culturing, serological or other techniques, and to call on the expertise and equipment of a specialist laboratory. These special techniques are not described here, but their use is briefly discussed.

Further reading

Crewe W. Laboratory diagnostic methods for parasitic diseases. In: Strickland GT (ed) *Hunter's Tropical Medicine*, 6th edn. Philadelphia, Saunders: 1984.

8

Examination of blood

The presence of protozoan and helminth parasites in blood is detected by micro-scopical examination of films of the blood. The specimen of blood for examina-tion is obtained by cleaning an area of skin with ether, alcohol or some similar fluid, and then pricking the cleaned area with a needle (or other instrument) that has a cutting edge and not a stabbing point. The drop of blood is touched with the surface of a clean, grease-free microscope slide, and when the slide is lifted away the blood is carried with it. Good preparations can be made only if the slide is scrupulously clean, and the simplest way to obtain such slides is to soak them for several hours in a hot solution of detergent and then rinse them in clean running water or water that is frequently changed. The slides can then be stored in clean boxes. After cleaning, the slides should be handled only by the edges; and scratched slides should never be used for making blood films.

Parasites that are intercellular, living in the plasma, may be observed (though not specifically identified) in a film of fresh blood — a 'wet' blood film. This is produced by placing a small drop of blood on the centre of a slide and then care-fully placing a coverslip on the drop. If the correct size of drop has been used, the blood will spread to the edges of the coverslip and form a layer which is one cell thick. Parasites such as microfilariae, trypanosomes and spirochaetes will reveal their presence under the low power (say × 100) of the microscope, because their movements jostle the surrounding red blood cells. They can usually be identified under higher magnification (say × 400).

Specific identification of parasites requires the preparation of dried and stained films. These are of two kinds: the 'thin' blood film in which the cells are discretely separated and flat, in a layer which is one cell thick, like the 'wet' blood film but now dried; and the 'thick' blood film, in which the blood cells are piled thickly and irregularly.

Thin blood films

A thin blood film is made by first placing a drop of blood near one end of a clean microscope slide. A 'spreader' slide, narrower than normal and usually made by cutting off the corner of a normal slide, is held touching the slide with the blood on it and at an angle of about 30° to the horizontal. The spreader slide is then drawn backwards until it touches the drop of blood, when the blood will run along the angle between the two slides. The spreader slide is then pushed forward with a deliberate steady movement, drawing the blood behind it to produce a film with straight edges. If the correct amount of blood has been used, the film will end in a series of 'tails' before it reaches the end of the slide. After it has been prepared, the film is dried by waving it in the air and is then stored in a covered container or with the blood facing downwards to prevent airborne contamination. In a humid atmosphere the blood should be dried by warming it slightly (by any convenient method) so that lysis of the cells does not occur.

In films prepared in this way the parasitized cells tend to roll to the edges or to be carried to the tails of the film, so these parts should be examined first. Haemoglobin is retained by fixation before or during the staining, so intracellular parasites appear framed by the blood cells.

Thick blood films

A thick blood film is made by placing two or three drops of blood near the centre of a microscope slide, and spreading them with a needle or with the corner of another slide into a circular or rectangular smear about 2 cm wide. The area covered will be determined by the amount of blood used, and it should be possible to read print or to see the numbers on a watch through the finished smear. The film should be spread quickly before fibrin is formed or auto-agglutination of the blood cells takes place.

After spreading, the film should be dried as quickly as possible but not heated above 37°C. While drying, it should be kept horizontal and protected from dust and insects. The dried film is opaque, and the haemoglobin must be removed so that the parasites can be seen by transmitted light. The film is therefore not fixed in alcohol, but is stained with an aqueous stain that lyses the blood while staining takes place. The outlines of the red blood cells cannot be seen in the stained film.

Labelling blood films

Probably the best method of labelling a film is by using a writing diamond to mark the slide with the patient's name, date, reference number, and any other information preferred. Thin films can be labelled, when dry, by writing on the film itself with a sharp graphite pencil or a needle.

Staining blood films

Many different variations of the original Romanowsky stain are now used in different parts of the world, and basically they are all mixtures of methylene blue and its oxidation products, the so-called azure dyes. In aqueous solution they stain the cytoplasm of parasites grey-blue and the chromatin reddish-purple. The stains most commonly used in Europe are Leishman's, Giemsa's and Field's, but others (which are just as effective) may be used in other continents.

Leishman's stain

Leishman's stain, which is an alcoholic solution, is used for thin blood films only. The stain can be bought already prepared or as a powder. In the latter case, the powder is dissolved in methyl alcohol according to the manufacturer's instructions, and the solution is ready for use 24 hours later, after it has been filtered.

For staining thin blood films, 0.5 ml of stain is placed on the horizontal slide with the blood film uppermost. This fixes the film in about 30 seconds. 1.5 ml of water, buffered at a pH of 7.2, is then added, and the mixture is then left for about 10 minutes for staining protozoa in blood (or about 15 minutes for staining *Leishmania* in tissue smears). The stain is then flooded off with running water as quickly as possible, and the slide is placed upright to dry. Prolonged washing should be avoided, otherwise the water-soluble methylene blue will be removed from the cytoplasm of the parasites very quickly.

Giemsa's stain

This stain can also be bought as a powder, but because preparation of the stain is complicated it is usually bought as a solution. Giemsa's stain is used after dilution in water, so it is suitable for use with thick blood films. It can also be used for staining thin blood films if these are fixed in alcohol for at least 30 seconds before they are stained. Thick films must not be fixed, otherwise the cells will not be lysed during the staining process and the film will be valueless.

The fixed thin films are stained for about 30 minutes in a 10 per cent solution of Giemsa's stain in buffered water (pH = 7.2). Thick films are stained for about 1 hour in a 3 per cent solution of stain in buffered water. These timings are not absolute, and various combinations of time and strength of stain have been used effectively.

After staining, the slides are washed rapidly and gently in water, and placed upright to dry.

Field's stain

This stain has the advantage, for clinical use, of being the most rapid, but it is suitable only for thick blood films. It consists of two solutions: solution A is essentially a solution of methylene blue and azure dyes in buffered water, and solution B is a mordant (usually eosin) solution in buffered water. The staining process also requires water with a pH of 7.0–7.2; buffered water is not necessary, and distilled water or clean tap water with the correct pH is satisfactory.

The thick blood film is lysed and stained simultaneously. The film is dipped in solution A for 5 seconds, washed gently in the water for 5 seconds, dipped in solution B for 3 seconds, and finally washed in the water for 5 seconds. Different parts of the film take up the stain to different degrees. The optimum staining of parasites occurs where the nuclei of the white blood cells are stained a reddish-purple, and this is usually somewhere near the edges of the film.

Protozoa, and particularly malaria parasites, in the blood are more easily seen and identified in thin blood films than in thick films. Thick films, however, have the important advantage of enabling the microscopist to examine much larger volumes of blood than is feasible with thin films, and so providing what is effectively a concentration of the parasites.

Staining of microfilariae

Microfilariae, the smallest of which is about 200 μm in length, can easily be seen in wet blood films. For specific identification, however, the arrangement of nuclei in the tail (see Fig. 7.3) has to be seen microscopically in stained thick blood films. The stains normally used are Mayer's acid haemalum and Giemsa's stain.

Meyer's acid haemalum is prepared by first dissolving 2 g of haematoxylin crystals in 10 ml of alcohol. 50 g of potassium aluminium sulphate is then dissolved in hot water, and to this solution is added the haematoxylin solution and also 0.2 g of sodium iodate. The resulting mixture is then made up to 1 litre with distilled water. The solution is then allowed to cool, and finally a crystal of thymol and 20 ml of glacial acetic acid are added.

The thick blood film is immersed in water until haemoglobin ceases to dissolve out; then it is dried in air and fixed in methyl alcohol for about 1 minute. The fixed film is dried in air again, then stained in hot (but not boiling) Mayer's haemalum for 5–10 minutes. The stain is washed off by immersing the slide in water, and the nuclei of the microfilariae become blue as the washing continues. The sheath of the microfilariae (if present) is stained as well as the nuclei.

Alternatively the blood film may be stained for 1 hour in a 3 per cent solution of Giemsa's stain in buffered water at a pH of 7.2. As the film has not been fixed, lysis of the cells and staining occur simultaneously. The film is then washed — carefully, because it is not fixed — and dried in air. Although the Romanowsky stains do not stain the sheath of a microfilaria as well as does haemalum, this technique is useful where both *Wuchereria bancrofti* and *Brugia malayi* are possibly present in the blood, because these species are stained differentially. Romanowsky-stained films have the additional advantage that they can also be used for the diagnosis of malaria.

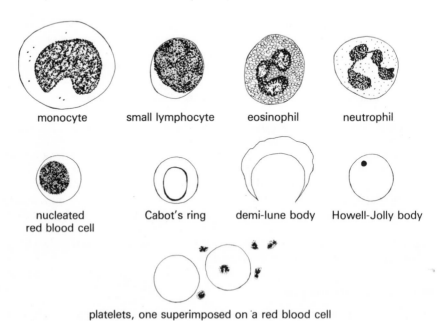

monocyte   small lymphocyte   eosinophil   neutrophil

nucleated   Cabot's ring   demi-lune body   Howell-Jolly body
red blood cell

platelets, one superimposed on a red blood cell

Fig. 8.1   Some constituents of blood that are frequently mistaken for parasites.

Artefacts

In a properly stained blood film, any parasites that are present have red or reddish-purple nuclei and blue or bluish-grey cytoplasm. Objects that do not show this differential staining are most unlikely to be parasites; and there are many objects in stained blood film that may be mistaken for parasites (Fig. 8.1).

Nucleated red blood cells are not uncommon, but the nucleus of one of these is dark and is the same colour all over. The nucleus may be broken, and may appear as small fragments (Howell–Jolly bodies) or rings (Cabot's rings), but the absence of a red nucleus indicates that these are not parasites. Platelets lying on red blood cells are often mistaken for parasites, as are contaminants from the air, from the solutions used in preparing the stains, and so on. If objects are found, apparently in red blood cells, which appear to be unidentified parasites, examination of the areas of the film between the blood cells will often reveal similar bodies and enable them to be identified as blood platelets, contaminants such as bacteria, or other non-parasitic bodies.

9

Examination of faeces

The presence of intestinal protozoa and worms is confirmed by the examination of specimens of faeces. The faeces should be passed into a clean container and not mixed with antiseptics or with urine. Examination of the faeces should be made as soon as possible after the specimen is passed.

Examination of the faeces should first be made macroscopically, to identify the presence of blood, mucus, or any worms or parts of worms; and it is often useful to note the general appearance of the specimen — for example, whether it is formed, loose or diarrhoeic, its colour, and its smell.

No technique is completely successful in detecting parasites by a single stool examination. Cysts are not regularly excreted but tend to appear in 'showers', and probably five or more consecutive stool specimens must be examined before an individual can be considered free from protozoal infections. In addition, both cysts and eggs may be present only in small numbers. There is no overall 'best' technique for detecting scanty parasites, although some techniques may be better than others in particular circumstances. The techniques described below are relatively simple, and should identify the presence of nearly all intestinal parasites unless they are present only in very small numbers.

Direct smears

The great majority of infections with intestinal protozoa and helminths are identified by examination of simple emulsions of faeces in physiological saline solution. To prepare such an emulsion, a drop of saline is placed on the centre of a microscope slide. With a small stick about the size of a match, or some similar implement, material is selected from several parts of the faecal specimen, including any blood or mucus present. About 2 mg (or 2 mm^3) of the material is rubbed on to the slide near the drop of saline, and then gradually mixed with the saline to form an even suspension. Any large particles of faeces are removed, and a coverslip is placed on the suspension carefully to avoid the formation of air bubbles. The finished preparation should be such that it is just possible to read print through it.

The entire area of the preparation should then be examined carefully and methodically under the lower power of the microscope (about × 100), and any objects that appear to be cysts or eggs should be examined under the dry high power (about × 400) to confirm the identification. Helminth eggs can be identified by their morphology: cysts cannot normally be specifically identified in saline preparations, but their shape and size can be determined.

Staining of faecal smears

Cysts of most of the intestinal protozoa, and especially those of the amoebae, require staining before they can be identified, and the stain most commonly used is a 1 per cent solution of iodine in potassium iodide. An emulsion of faeces is prepared in the same way as described above, except that the iodine solution is used instead of physiological saline. The protozoan cysts stain progressively with the iodine, and after a suitable period (usually about 5 minutes) the nuclei can be seen and counted.

Concentration of cysts and eggs

When cysts or eggs are present only in very small numbers, it may be necessary to carry out some form of concentration in order to recognize the infection. There are many techniques for concentrating the parasites in faeces, some designed for particular parasites; and essentially these can be divided into flotation techniques, in which the eggs or cysts are lifted away from heavier debris, and sedimentation techniques, in which the eggs sink to the bottom of a container while the lighter debris floats. Details of various techniques are given in the appropriate textbooks, but examples of useful methods are given below.

Zinc sulphate flotation

This technique is suitable for the concentration of cysts, and of eggs other than those of the trematodes. Trematode eggs are operculated, and so they burst and become unidentifiable in a hypertonic solution.

The zinc sulphate solution is prepared by dissolving 331 g of zinc sulphate crystals in 1 litre of water. The specific gravity of the solution should be checked with a hydrometer to ensure that it is 1.18. About 1 g of the faeces is emulsified in water, and strained through a fine wire or nylon sieve into a 15 ml centrifuge tube. This is centrifuged at 250–350g for 2 minutes, the supernatant fluid is decanted, fresh water is added and the tube is shaken. This procedure is repeated until the supernatant fluid remains clear. The clear supernatant fluid is then discarded, and the tube is filled to half-way with the zinc sulphate solution of specific gravity 1.18. The tube is shaken, and more zinc sulphate is added to fill the tube to within 5 mm of the brim. The tube is then centrifuged at 600 g for 1 minute, and the surface scum is transferred by means of a wire loop to a microscope slide, and covered with a coverslip. The preparation is then examined under the microscope, after staining with iodine if necessary. Alternatively, with the addition of another step and instead of transferring the surface material by a loop, the top 3 ml of the supernatant fluid can be pipetted into a clean centrifuge tube. This tube is filled with water, shaken, and centrifuged, and the deposit is transferred to a microscope slide and examined microscopically.

Sodium chloride flotation

This is a simple method of concentration, and is useful for the examination of faeces for eggs of *Ascaris* or hookworms. A small amount of the faeces, about 1–2 mm^3, is emulsified in about 10 ml of a saturated solution of sodium chloride and strained through a fine wire or nylon sieve. The sieved mixture is then placed in a straight-walled tube about 7.5 cm high, and the tube is filled with saturated sodium chloride until a menicus is formed above the brim of the tube. A cover-slip is then placed on the meniscus, and the tube is left for 20 minutes. After this time the coverslip is removed with a straight upward lift, placed on a microscope slide, and examined with a magnification of about × 100 for eggs.

Other flotation techniques involve the use of solutions of salts such as sodium nitrate, zinc chloride and magnesium sulphate, with specific gravities adjusted to float the eggs being looked after.

Sedimentation in water

This is a simple technique, and is useful for many parasites other than schisto-somes, the eggs of which hatch in water. The faeces are rubbed through a wire or nylon sieve into water to produce a thin suspension, which is placed in a conical urine glass. The material is left to settle, the supernatant liquid is poured away, and the glass is refilled with water. This changing of the supernatant liquid is repeated at intervals of not less than 1 hour until the supernatant liquid remains clear. This clear supernatant liquid is then discarded, and the sediment is examined microscopically for eggs and cysts.

If schistosome eggs are thought to be present, the sedimentation should be carried out not in water but in physiological saline or in a 0.5 per cent solution of glycerine.

Formol—ether sedimentation

This is probably the most useful 'general' technique for the concentration of parasites from faeces. It concentrates helminth larvae and eggs, and protozoan cysts, and can be used for fresh specimens or for specimens that have been collected and then preserved in formalin. The technique is as follows.

Approximately 1 g of faeces is emulsified in about 10 ml of water, and the mixture is sieved through a wire or nylon sieve into a 15 ml centrifuge tube. The tube is centrifuged at about 350 g for 2 minutes, the supernatant fluid is discarded, the tube is refilled with water, and then centrifuged again. This is repeated until the supernatant fluid remains clear. The clear supernatant fluid is then discarded, and 10 ml of formol saline and 3 ml of ether are added to the sediment. The tube is shaken vigorously and centrifuged with the speed being regulated so that the centrifugal force reaches 600 g after 2 minutes. The centrifuge is then switched off, and allowed to come to rest without braking.

The tube will now show an upper layer of ether and a lower layer of formol saline, and at the interface between the two liquids will be a layer of debris. This debris is loosened with a swab stick, and the whole of the supernatant liquid is poured away with the layer of debris. The remaining deposit in the tube is shaken up with the small drop of fluid in the bottom of the centrifuge tube, then transferred to a microscope slide and covered with a coverslip. This preparation is then examined under a microscope, after staining with 1 per cent iodine if necessary.

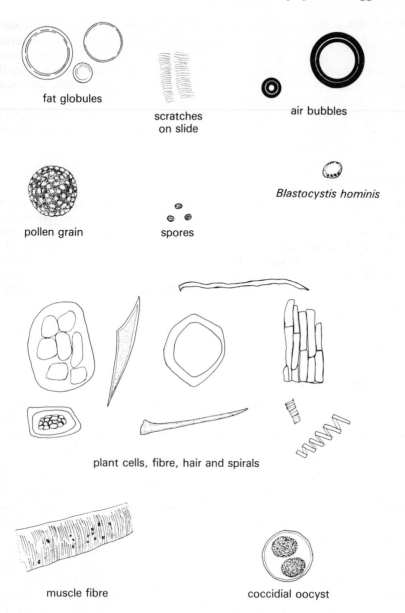

fat globules

scratches
on slide

air bubbles

pollen grain

spores

Blastocystis hominis

plant cells, fibre, hair and spirals

muscle fibre

coccidial oocyst

Fig. 9.1   Some constituents of faeces that are frequently mistaken for parasites.

Artefacts

Various objects that somehow resemble parasites or stages of parasites may frequently be seen in preparations of faeces (Fig. 9.1). Small spherical bodies which may be amoebic cysts should be examined under a magnification of about × 400. Amoebic cysts, and indeed cysts of any of the intestinal protozoa, have very thin walls which can be sharply focussed, and they are all approximately the same size. Plant cells, on the other hand, have thick walls which vary in thickness in different parts; and fat globules, oil droplets and air bubbles cannot be sharply focussed, and vary greatly in size in the same specimen. Finally, any object that is coloured in an unstained faecal smear cannot be a protozoan cyst.

Eggs of helminth parasites nearly always have a smooth outline (Fig. 9.2), and bodies that are roughly oval but irregularly shaped are usually plant cells. Helminth larvae are usually active in faecal smears unless chemicals have been added. Even if they are motionless they can be recognized by the structure of the intestine, and by the fact that they are more or less pointed at each end. Plant hairs have one flat end where they have been broken off the plant.

It should always be borne in mind that under the low power of the microscope it is not usually possible to do more than tentatively identify an object as parasitic. It is necessary to examine the object under a higher magnification to decide whether it is a parasite, and to identify it positively.

Fig. 9.2 Eggs of Helminth parasites of Man.
a. *Clonorchis* group; b. *Taenia*; c. *Hymenolepis*; d. *Trichuris*; e. *Enterobius*; f. *Ascaris* (fertile); g. *Ascaris* (decorticated); h. Hookworm; j. *Diphyllobothrium*; k. *Ascaris* (infertile); l. *Schistosoma japonicum*; m. *Paragonimus*; n. *Schistosoma haematobium*; o. *Schistosoma mansoni*; p. *Fasciola* or *Fasciolopsis*.

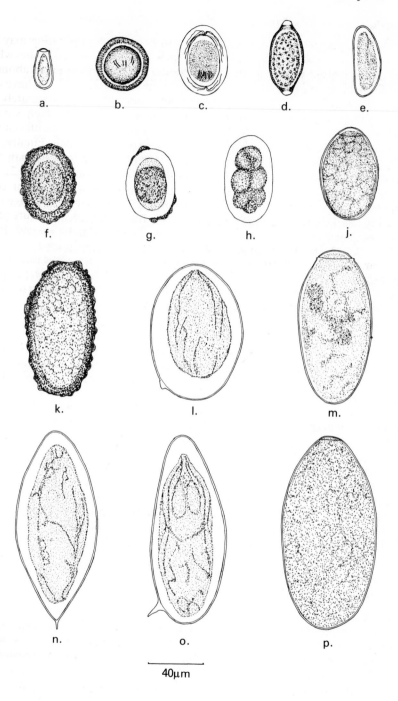

40μm

10

Examination of other specimens

Although identification of the great majority of parasites found in man is made by examining preparations of blood or faeces, it is also possible to find adult or immature stages of parasites in urine, sputum and cerebrospinal fluid, in tissue exudates, aspirates and biopsies, and occasionally in other specimens. Examination of specimens other than blood or faeces may be the usual way of identifying infection, as by examination of skin biopsies for onchocerciasis, or a very important ancillary method of diagnosis, as by examination of cerebrospinal fluid for African trypanosomiasis. However, as these techniques are used relatively rarely, they will be discussed here only briefly. If full details of the various techniques are required, they can be found in textbooks on clinical laboratory diagnosis.

Urine

Urine is usually examined to detect eggs of schistosomes, particularly those of *S. haematobium*. The urine should if possible be collected between 11 a.m. and 2 p.m., as this is the peak time for excretion of eggs, and the whole specimen allowed to stand for about 30 minutes in a conical urine glass. After this interval the sediment is collected with a pipette, placed on a microscope slide, and examined under the microscope for eggs. A rapid and very sensitive (though not simple) technique using Nuclepore filters has been described, but it is used mainly for quantitative work.

In infections with *Wuchereria bancrofti*, where there is chyluria, microfilariae may be discharged in the urine. To look for microfilariae, the urine is centrifuged at high speed, the supernatant fluid is discarded, and the sediment is collected with a pipette and examined under the microscope. Any microfilariae present will be alive, and can be easily identified by their active movements. The specimen can be dried, fixed in alcohol, and stained in the same way as a blood film for identification of the microfilariae.

Sputum

Rupture of a pulmonary abscess may result in the coughing up of some of its contents, including trophozoites of *Entamoeba histolytica*, and rupture of a pulmonary hydatid cyst may similarly result in the coughing up of protoscoleces of *Echinococcus granulosus*. Sputum may also contain eggs of *Paragonimus* or migrating larval nematodes.

If the sputum contains pus and amoebiasis is suspected, a freshly produced specimen should be examined directly for trophozoites, keeping it at 37°C during the examination. For other parasites, the sputum should be thoroughly mixed with an equal volume of a 3 per cent solution of sodium hydroxide and either allowed to sediment or centrifuged at 1400 *g* for 30 minutes. The deposit is then transferred to a microscope slide and examined microscopically for eggs of *Paragonimus* or stages of other parasites.

Aspirates

Both protozoa and helminths may be found in aspirated material from various organs. Aspirates from the small intestine may be obtained by a nasogastric tube, or by the 'Entero-test' in which the patient swallows a weighted length of nylon string. The weight passes into the duodenum, and 4 hours or more afterwards the string is withdrawn by a gentle steady pull and examined for parasites, particularly *Giardia* and *Strongyloides*, which may not have shown signs of their presence in the faeces.

Aspirations from liver and lung abscesses can be examined for trophozoites of *E. histolytica*; and material from lymph nodes, liver, bone marrow and voluntary muscle may be of help in the diagnosis of African trypanosomiasis, visceral leishmaniasis and American trypanosomiasis. Aspirates in suspected cases of African trypanosomiasis are examined directly for motile trypanosomes, or they may be smeared, fixed in alcohol, and stained with one of the Romanowsky stains. Aspirates in cases of visceral leishmaniasis may be cultured, or prepared as fixed and suitably stained smears.

Biopsies

Skin-inhabiting microfilariae may be identified by the examination of skin 'snips'. The skin surface is first cleaned with alcohol or ether, and a small piece of skin is lifted with the point of a fine needle. The skin attached to the needle is then cut off with a safety-razor blade, which is held horizontally and moved towards the needle — the skin is cut just below the point of the needle, so that no blood is drawn. The small piece of skin is then placed in a drop of physiological saline in a cavity slide, and examined under the microscope. Any microfilariae present will emerge from the skin snip, and after about 30 minutes most of them will be visible moving in the saline. If required, the preparation can be allowed to dry, fixed, and then stained in the same way as a blood film for identification of the microfilariae. Skin biopsies or skin scrapings may also be used to identify the causes of ulcers and other lesions on the body surface.

Muscle biopsy may assist in the diagnosis of trichinosis, but it is not reliable. A small portion of muscle is removed, squeezed between two glass plates, and either examined directly for larvae under the low power of the microscope (× 100), or digested in artificial gastric juice at 37°C and the living larvae which are released concentrated by centrifuging. Muscle biopsy may also be used to assist in the identification of macroscopic bodies such as larvae of cestodes.

Biopsy of the large intestine or bladder, by means of a proctoscope, sigmoidoscope or cystoscope, is sometimes of value in infections with schistosomes. The piece of mucous membrane can be pressed between glass plates and examined for schistosome eggs under the low power (× 100) of the microscope.

11

Immunodiagnosis of parasitic infections

Specific diagnosis of parasitic infections is most satisfactorily achieved by identification of parasites or their developmental stages in excreta, body fluids or tissues. Detection of antibodies or a positive skin test is less specific as an index of active infection, for these findings may indicate past rather than present parasitization. Detection of immunoglobulin M antibody is sometimes helpful in diagnosing current infection, as for example in toxoplasmosis. Serological diagnosis has also been unsatisfactory because lack of specificity of antigens can give rise to cross-reactions between parasites, especially helminths. The use of hybridoma technology is enabling the preparation of more specific monoclonal antigens, and this may overcome problems associated with poor specificity. These techniques may also make antigen detection possible; and the presence of antigen is indicative of active infection. Antigen detection has already been achieved in malaria.

Identification of parasites or their products is difficult in some conditions,

Table 11.1 Serological tests in parasitic diseases

Serological test	Reactivity	Parasitic diseases in which the test is useful
Complement fixation (CFT)	Low	American trypanosomiasis; echinococcosis; pneumocystosis; paragonimiasis; cyticercosis
Indirect immunofluorescence (IFAT)	Medium	American and African trypanosomiasis; filariasis; leishmaniasis; malaria; toxoplasmosis; schistosomiasis
Indirect haemagglutination (IHA)	Medium	Amoebiasis; echinococcosis; stronglyloidiasis; filariasis; toxoplasmosis; cysticercosis
Agglutination	Low	Leishmaniasis
Enzyme-linked immunosorbent assay (ELISA)	High	Toxocariasis; toxoplasmosis; leishmaniasis; schistosomiasis
Latex agglutination (LAT)	Low	Amoebiasis
Bentonite flocculation tests (BFT)	Low	Trichinosis

such as amoebic liver abscess, toxoplasmosis, hydatid disease and cysticercosis. It is in such conditions that serological diagnosis is useful. Serological methods are also useful in epidemiological surveys of populations.

Table 11.2 Assessment of serological tests

Condition	Tests	Remarks
Amoebic liver abscess	IHA; LAT; IFAT	Serological tests positive in 95% of cases of ALA; trophozoites difficult to find in abscess aspirates
American trypanosomiasis	CFT; IHA; IFAT	Trypanosomes difficult to detect in chronic cases; sensitivity good and specificity fair (some cross-reactions with leishmaniasis); useful for screening blood for transfusion
Cutaneous leishmaniasis	IFAT; IHA	Parasites may be scanty in lesions; Leishmanin skin test helpful
Visceral leishmaniasis	CCIE*	Serology a useful screening test; Leishmanin test negative until cured
Toxoplasmosis	Dye test; IFAT; specific IgM detection	Parasites very difficult to obtain from lesions or blood; detection of specific IgM denotes recent infection — important in pregnancy
Hydatid disease	CFT; LAT; Casoni skin test	Cyst aspiration contraindicated; tests reasonably specific and sensitive; Casoni test is sensitive but not specific, and outmoded
Cysticercosis	CFT; IHA	Helpful in cerebral disease; sensitivity low in chronic disease
Occult filariasis; filarial elephantiasis	ELISA; IFAT; immunoelectrophoresis	Microfilària absent from blood in these conditions
Toxocariasis	ELISA; agar gel diffusion	ELISA specific and sensitive in visceral larva migrans, but often negative in retinal lesions
Trichinosis	IFAT; CFT; BFT	Serology can be diagnostic but usually not for 3–4 weeks after onset of illness
African trypanosomiasis	IFAT; ELISA; card agglutination; IgM levels	Useful; trypomastigotes often not found in blood or CSF; card agglutination can be performed in the field; high IgM indicates need for specific tests.

* CCIE = counter current immunoelectrophoresis

Table 11.3 Conditions in which serological diagnosis is of limited value

Malaria	Serological tests for malaria such as IFAT, ELISA and IHA are of little use in the diagnosis of individual cases of acute malaria. The techniques have applications in monitoring the persistence of the disease during control programmes, and in confirming or refuting the diagnosis in individuals who claim to have recurrent attacks of fever due to malaria.
Schistosomiasis	Specific chemotherapy of schistosomiasis is only indicated when living eggs are found in the excreta, or when there are suspected CNS lesions. Positive serology alone is not an indication for treatment. Contact with animal or bird schistosomes is not uncommon and can produce false positives. Serology may remain positive for years after cure. Serology can be useful in the diagnosis of Katayama fever and neurological schistosomiasis when eggs may not be found in the excreta. IFAT and ELISA tests are now being used for diagnosis with some success.
Pneumocystis carinii	These protozoa are difficult to isolate from the respiratory tract. Unfortunately serology using the IFAT and CFT is not very helpful, for the tests are not highly sensitive and many healthy adults and children have antibodies as a result of previous infection.
Intestinal, biliary and lung fluke infections	In these infections the eggs can usually be found in faeces or sputum. In paragonimiasis and fascioliasis eggs may be difficult to find, and in these infections serology may be helpful.

Serological techniques in use

Many of the immunological techniques used in bacterial disease are also used in parasitic disease. Some of these are shown in Table 11.1. Many laboratories are able to carry out some, but not all, of these tests for routine diagnosis.

An ideal test would have high specificity (very few false positives), high sensitivity (very few false negatives) and high reactivity (able to detect very small quantities of antigen). Skin tests usually detect cell-mediated immunity or reaginic activity, and they are not widely used in parasitology because of their low specificity. Nevertheless, the Leishmanin skin test is valuable in the diagnosis of cutaneous leishmaniasis.

Conditions in which serological tests are of considerable use in diagnosis are shown in Table 11.2, and those in which the tests are of limited value are shown in Table 11.3.

Further reading

Cohen S, Warren KS. *Immunology of Parasitic Infections*, 2nd ed. Oxford: Blackwell Scientific Publications, 1982.

Houba V. *Immunological Investigation of Tropical Diseases*. Edinburgh: Churchill Livingstone, 1980.

Kagan IG. Serodiagnosis and Skin tests. In: Strickland GT (ed) *Hunter's Tropical Medicine*, 6th edn. Philadelphia, Saunders: 1005–10, 1984.

Wakelin D. *Immunity to parasites*. London, Arnold: 1984.

Index